The
Psychiatric Hospital
as a
Therapeutic
Instrument

The Psychiatric Hospital as a Therapeutic Instrument

Collected Papers of High Point Hospital

Edited by
ALEXANDER GRALNICK, M.D.
Medical Director, High Point Hospital
Associate Clinical Professor of Psychiatry,
New York Medical College

BRUNNER/MAZEL, *Publishers* • New York • 1969

Published by
BRUNNER/MAZEL, INC.
80 East 11th Street
New York, N. Y. 10003

Library of Congress Catalog Card No. 75-77585

SBN 87630-012-3

MANUFACTURED IN THE UNITED STATES OF AMERICA

TO THE MEMORY OF

WILLIAM V. SILVERBERG, M.D.

Teacher, Colleague, Counselor and
Good Friend

Preface

MANY AND ALWAYS INCREASING in number are the psychiatric therapeutic approaches; still, hospital treatment remains the therapy of choice for a large group of patients.

The psychiatric hospital has repeatedly changed status and acquired different images. At first it was a place relegated to custodial care; then it became a sanitarium where predominantly physical therapies were administered. In a third period of time it became a place where individual psychotherapy and milieu therapy achieved a prominent role. In the fourth and present stage the modern hospital has acquired, in addition to the roles already mentioned, a key position in the rapidly expanding community psychiatry.

In the third and fourth stages High Point Hospital has acquired and maintains a high point of leadership. The collection of papers presented in this volume reveals that this leadership is actualized not only in the practical care of the patient, but also in research and scholarship.

The problems inherent in hospital treatment are many and intricate. On one side the hospital is an environment where a group of people have to be taken care of under collective rule; and on the other side, it is a place where the person has to be recognized and accepted in his own individuality and treated according to his specific requirements. The hospital is a place where certain limitations and structured activities are required by the psychological status of the patients, and yet it must be a place where an atmosphere of freedom and warm understanding is offered. The psychiatric hospital is a center where the family of the patient is guided to change its role, and, at the same time, it is a place where the family is studied, evaluated, appreciated, cultivated, informed, and instructed, so that its influence on the patient will be a favorable one after his hospitalization. At the same time that the hospital represents a protective barrier between the patient and the community, it must break down this very barrier. By decreasing the differences between its own environment and that of the outside world, and by increasing its interaction with society, the modern psychiatric hospital reduces the traditional isolation and assumes a new role in the community. Hospitalization no longer needs to be an additional psychological trauma to the already severely traumatized patient; nor does it need to foster dependency. Together with various forms of rehabilitation of the patient, it enhances in him a feeling of more and more intense participation in the group and in life in general.

This collection of papers reveals how some of these problems, seeming paradoxes and dichotomies, are solved at High Point Hospital and can be solved elsewhere.

Silvano Arieti, M.D.

Clinical Professor of Psychiatry
New York Medical College

Foreword

High Point Hospital is a forty-five bed psychiatric institution located in an idyllic setting on the outskirts of a suburb of New York City. From the outside it has the physical appearance of any one of a number of small proprietary mental hospitals or sanitaria scattered in semi-rural areas of the United States, suggesting that it follows the traditional model for such institutions, i.e. conscientiously doing what is possible with a limited staff who use a variety of modalities of treatment to guide patients toward restitution. Yet in actuality High Point Hospital presents a totally different image of a proprietary mental hospital and this publication dedicates itself to that difference. It demonstrates how a psychiatric hospital by virtue of its organized and yet fluent structure and programs can be an *instrument in therapy*.

The hospital opened its doors in 1951 on the initiative of Dr. Alexander Gralnick. His own background in clinical psychiatry and psychoanalysis determined the operational model for the institution. Psychoanalytically-oriented psychotherapy, both as a treatment method and as an attitude, was from the beginning its very substance. The early papers on psychotherapy and on concepts of psychoanalysis in connection with inpatients, some of which are published in this volume, reflect the immediacy of this predilection. But Gralnick is a combination of psychiatric clinician, psychoanalyst, and administrator endowed with an indefatigable drive for work of high standard and a will to inspire those who work with him to do likewise. He has these objectives: to make his hospital second to none; to give it a university atmosphere in training and research knowing that this enhances patient care; to push forward the frontiers of knowledge concerning the hospitalized patient; and to change the image of the proprietary hospital. This volume with its twenty papers selected from the many published by the staff between 1954 and 1968 is one example of how he succeeded.

In a demostration to establish the hospital in the foreground of psychiatric theory and practice Gralnick and his co-workers began to explore parameters in research vogue at the time, such as milieu therapy, the therapeutic community, family therapy, and social psychiatry. But they were distinctly not dealing with clichés, psychiatric fashions, or "on the bandwagon" exercises. Because of the special characteristics of the hospital, its small patient population, large staff, policies of extended care, and particular philosophy, it brought to the concepts of milieu and family therapy a special idea.

This occurred as a result of the highly refined system of clinical administration which worked so effectively that it could be controlled for use as a therapeutic instrument or agent as indicated. The practice of acknowledging every detail, no matter how small, as a possible stimulus for meaningful interaction served as a gyroscope for the social structure of a psychiatric setting and provided additional sources of raw data. The use of clinical administration as if it were a sensitive instrument, like radar, to guide the psychotherapeutic milieu encompassing patients, their families, and staff through emotional and social vicissitudes toward a controlled environment which effects optimal healing is the essence of the papers in this volume.

It is pleasing to contemplate that the power of this little giant, working apart from a university and medical school with a relatively small number of subjects over an extended period of time, may have succeeded in distilling for psychiatry purer research elements and results than may be possible in more complex environments. This contribution of a controlled environment which continuously dares to evaluate itself is refreshing for psychiatry. And from these papers one may learn how it can be done.

At this point in the development of psychiatric theory and practice, many clinical units are cognizant of the issues described here and are investigating them as all-important elements in inpatient psychiatry. The special contribution of High Point Hospital to this body of knowledge will, I am certain, prove to be a valuable one.

MAURICE H. GREENHILL, M.D.

Professor of Psychiatry
Albert Einstein College of Medicine

Contents

Page

Introduction

THOUGH THE MANY CURRENTS in psychiatry will come to bear on any institution, ultimately it will develop its own theme. This theme, in turn, will be a reflection of some aspect of the general scene in psychiatry of which the hospital is perforce a part. At the same time, the life history of a psychiatric hospital is unique, and the experience its staff brings to it will determine whether its primary emphasis will be on the physical therapies or milieu and psychotherapy. The philosophy and values of those who determine the hospital's destiny will also define its social structure, which, in turn, will have an essential bearing on the therapeutic results.

Considering their training background, it was inevitable that the founders of High Point Hospital should emphasize psychotherapy, family and milieu therapy, and eventually the psychotherapeutic-community as a therapeutic instrument. It was logical too that their main research efforts should be clinical and devoted to the study of the patient in action, in interaction and in relation to his social environment, that is, social psychiatry. The included papers culled from our publications mirror the thinking of our Hospital's Staff, and trace the development of its therapeutic approach. It is hoped that, read in succession or as they were written chronologically, they will adequately present the concept of the psychiatric hospital as a therapeutic instrument—an organization of people consistently functioning in unison, with commonly accepted psychiatric methods, goals, policies and values. The psychiatric hospital acting as a therapeutic instrument is not a mere collection of factors, nor is it noted for any single aspect of its program. It is always in action as a total unit.

This book will have principal appeal for those who believe mental illness is rooted in the patient's life experience. However, it is hoped that the papers will also be of interest to our organically-oriented colleagues, if only as a clear exposition of how those "on the other side" view and treat the mentally ill. It is intended, further, that this book will demonstrate why and how the analytically-trained psychiatrist modifies his theories and practices in the fires of clinical experience with the hospitalized patient. There is a vast difference between the office and hospital practice of psychiatry, and on this account it is also hoped that the book will be of interest to the practitioner in both areas.

At any instant a "hospital" is the culmination of the efforts of those—patients and staff alike—who have passed through its doors. Thus, the ideas expressed in this book have been gleaned from all of these people. Although the individual authors brought their own creative talents to the scene, they also express the substance of the hospital environment in which they found themselves immersed. This volume then is the end-result of a total effort of many, but at the same time, a representation of its several authors. The editor acknowledges with much thanks the special efforts of the respective authors, and expresses his particular indebtedness to them for their assistance in his own growth and the development of ideas expressed by him herein.

I also wish to express my appreciation to the Board of Directors of our Hospital for its constant support and guidance and to Fanny Holmes, my secretary, for her faithful work on all the manuscripts. I am also indebted to the publishers of the various journals and books who permitted the reprinting of the papers which compose this volume.

ALEXANDER GRALNICK, M.D.

April, 1969
Port Chester, New York

The Psychiatric Hospital as a Therapeutic Instrument

1

Psychotherapy in a Private Mental Hospital

ALEXANDER GRALNICK, M.D.
MERVYN SCHACHT, M.D.
STEPHEN W. KEMPSTER, M.D.

WHEN DR. GUTHEIL CALLED to ask me if I would speak on the above subject, I felt hardly prepared. I was thinking in terms of clinical reports requiring many years of work. Dr. Gutheil, however, pointed out that you would probably be more interested in knowing about the organization of a hospital devoted to psychotherapy, the problems we encounter, the kinds of cases we handle, and ways we handle them. He suggested that you would want to know how such a hospital may help a patient, and how it functions to help the practicing therapist Is there anything, for instance, about such a hospital that could allay the misgivings a psychotherapist has about hospitalizing a patient? Must hospitalization be a traumatic experience, a waste of time from the psychotherapeutic point of view and need it result in a permanent severance of the therapeutic relationship?

I readily consented to prepare such a paper, and am very happy now that I did. I said at the time that I probably could stand up at a moment's notice and talk about such things several hours on end. I see now, however, that any

---

Reprinted from *American Journal of Psychotherapy,* Vol. VIII, No. 2, pp. 312-325. April, 1954. Read before the Association for the Advancement of Psychotherapy on March 27, 1953.

such extemporaneous attempt on my part would be better entitled "The Trials and Tribulations of Founding, Organizing and Running a Psychiatric Hospital"—or, as I sometimes feel, "Poor me!" What will follow instead will be in keeping with the title, "Psychotherapy in a Private Mental Hospital." I should like to say at the outset that this paper is largely the result of a joint effort on the part of myself as administrator and director, and Doctors Mervyn Schacht and Stephen Kempster, our very able attending psychotherapists.

Essentially, then, the facts as we see them and the thoughts presented, reflect the joint endeavor of the administrative and clinical personnel.

The subject of the evening evokes two quick questions: First, what is a private mental hospital? Second, what is psychotherapy?

I have posed these rather simple questions at the risk of being considered quite elementary, but, I believe, with good reason. We all have a more or less similar conception of the hospital as a public institution. It is generally a picture of a large number of patients, of overcrowded, large buildings, back wards, lack of individual attention, uniformity of treatment, rigidity of approach, doctors struggling to keep up with their work, and the like.

When we speak of the private hospital, we associate with it a variety of pictures. There is a lack of uniformity, based not so much on the fee-scale, as on many other factors. Among these are the aims of those who direct the hospital, their training and beliefs, the kinds of patients they admit, and the physical aspects of the hospital itself.

Where mental illness is considered a physiological process, the shock therapies will tend naturally to be emphasized. If one believes that "getting away from it all" is therapeutic in itself, one is more likely to organize a peaceful sort of hide-away. If one is of the opinion that concentration on one's self is bad, the hospital program may revolve about an organized occupational and recreational activity designed to divert the patient from his problems.

Probably no private program is pure in its culture, because most of us believe that many things enter into the curative process. Particularly today, when the emphasis on psychotherapy is increasing, and the long-term results of shock therapy prove to be rather disappointing, no one can afford to neglect psychotherapy entirely. As a result, a little bit of psychotherapy gets mixed into most of the programs of the private mental hospital.

Where those who run an institution have a variety of beliefs, or are scientifically inclined, a combination of approaches may be used, and one or the other treatment will be emphasized. There is no doubt, however, that a particular treatment procedure is usually believed to be most effective, and this takes precedence over all others. It is this one procedure, which, as a rule, determines the prevailing policy and is the core of the overall program.

In size, the private hospitals divide themselves roughly into the relatively large and small. The larger of these types are usually composed of numerous buildings and care for all kinds of patients in all the adult age groups. The ones I have in mind are long established, highly organized, and possess rather elaborate occupational and recreational activity programs, which are emphasized along with the conventional physiological therapies. Psychotherapy is part of the program, but is not considered of paramount importance. It suffers on three scores: (1) that it is not analytically oriented nor well supervised, (2) that it cannot be carried out on an intensive basis because of the low ratio between psychiatrist and patient, and (3) that because of the very size of the hospital, it cannot be associated with a rather individualized patient program.

The bulk of small private sanitaria are either custodial in nature, or they emphasize especially the physiologic therapies. Psychotherapy, while given more extensively than in the large private hospitals, is not necessarily applied with emphasis, and usually is considered as incidental or adjunctive to the shock treatments. The small private sanitaria devoted to psychotherapy as the keystone of their therapeutic program to which all other forms of therapy are subordinated are very few indeed.[1]

Before proceeding to a more detailed description of the private hospital devoted to psychotherapy, I should like to say a few words in response to the second question, namely, "What is psychotherapy?"

I think we all agree that psychotherapy is a process taking place between a therapist and patient and carried on by verbal communication, with the aim of furnishing the patient with insights which may help him to get well. With this as a basis, we would all agree on the following: First, that mental illness has a genesis, and that psychotherapy is directed towards uncovering it. Second, that traumatic incidents play a major role in causing mental disturbances, and that psychotherapy is directed toward unearthing and overcoming their effects. Third, that on the part of the patient there is unawareness of motivations, and that psychotherapy is directed toward furnishing awareness. Fourth, that in mental illness the nature of one's interpersonal relationships, both past and present, is of extreme significance, and that by means of psychotherapy such relationships can be understood and adjusted. Fifth, that there are social pressures which cause mental disturbances, and that psychotherapy is directed toward clarifying these. Sixth, that there are psycho-dynamic forces at play in the therapeutic relationship which psychotherapy studies and utilizes. Seventh, that there are psychological resistances to insight which psychotherapy aims to overcome.

We now come to a more specific description of the hospital devoted to psychotherapy. Nowhere is it more true than in the psychotherapy of hospitalized patients that treatment

---

[1] Frieda Fromm-Reichmann mentions six such in the world, and among them, High Point Hospital (*Specialized Techniques in Psychotherapy*, edited by Gustav Bychowski).

may founder at any moment. It is particularly necessary, therefore, to establish an atmosphere and an organization that will minimize the chance of failure, and offer the psychotherapist the best opportunity to carry on. Through the organization of the therapeutic facilities, one must furnish a fertile soil for the psychotherapeutic process to develop satisfactorily. This means the creation of an atmosphere which permits the expression of the unhealthy behavior so that it may be scrutinized for insights that will ultimately eradicate it. The atmosphere of a psychotherapeutic hospital must also promote new and healthier modes of behavior, motivations and attitudes. However, it may not injudiciously permit a behavior which is contrary to the patient's own welfare and that of those about him; while protective, it cannot be unduly restrictive.

Such a hospital must be flexible—close to the point of danger sometimes—if therapeutic progress is to be made. There are times when legal or family pressures, or the weight of tradition, must be fought—times when one is moving in the dark, and calculated risks must be taken. There must, on the other hand, be an air of quiet rule and regulation which the patients can accept as either fair and equitable or, at least, tolerable.

While flexibility must be maintained, it should not reach the point where chaos threatens. We have seen this happen on occasion, when too many patients were given too much leeway. This is likely to happen when one tries to meet the irrational demands of several patients without thought for the effect it may have on the rest of the group. The individual patient will frequently press for the satisfaction of his own demands, and if one relents to such pressure beyond the point of reason, neither the patient nor his fellow patients will benefit. At the same time, the group may be required to tolerate the egoistic behavior of the individual patient. The balance is often very delicate, and it may be difficult occasionally to draw the line properly. But this, to a large extent, is the work of the administrative-therapeutic team.

The medical and nursing personnel must exercise their authority with extreme judiciousness. They must be flexible but not weak, firm but not aggressive, They must be strong enough to enforce their decisions even in the face of hostility displayed by the individual patient or a group of patients. There should be authority without authoritarianism. At all times, however, authority must be tempered by the ability to retreat without rancor in the face of too explosive a situation; but it also must be resilient enough to return to the problem at a more propitious time. Those in authority must remember that it is not the winning or the losing of the battle with the patients which is of importance; the essential is that, as a result of the struggle, the patients should come out with more insight and the authorities with more knowledge.

Some people believe that a hospital should be a retreat from the world. In an institution devoted to psychotherapy, this can hardly be so, except in a limited sense. The patient who comes to our hospital with such a belief experiences some disappointment, for he soon finds he is in a rather well-organized, little society which will not relent to his morbid forms of behavior. Such a patient will have a rather difficult period of adjustment; sometimes he may even become quite upset, until his own better judgment prevails and the therapist's work can begin to bear fruit.

The overly-dependent patient who expects that the hospital will furnish inordinate amounts of support will also suffer some disappointment. Such a patient will suffer until the forces of the hospital can be mobilized to meet a modest amount of his dependency needs, and the therapist can help him overcome his extreme dependency. It is often feared that the extremely dependent patient may suffer as a result of hospitalization and that he may be using the institution as a haven and a permanent retreat. Such a possibility exists indeed; it can, however, be handled by the alert therapist who has an opportunity to approach it psychologically, and also by the hospital personnel and the patient's family, who can be mobilized to aid in combating this morbid tendency on the part of the patient. The "reality factor" of the financial expense involved often also counteracts such inclinations.

Instead of escaping the pressures of a domineering parent or marital partner, the struggle against competitive siblings, or the pressures of an authoritarian figure, the patient finds himself in a social situation peopled with similar figures, and charged with the same upsetting forces he has met in his everyday life. These may be the Director of the Hospital, a figure of authority and all that goes with it for the patient, the Directress of Nursing, who plays a significant role in the hospital, and the therapist himself, who may be seen as all manner of people, and exert all sorts of influences on the patient. He will find patients who will compete with him for the therapist's favors, and also reject his every overture.

Much of what I have been saying about the general atmosphere and the attitudes which necessarily prevail in a hospital devoted to psychotherapy hold for High Point Hospital, which cares for a variety of patients suffering from all sorts and degrees of mental illness.

When we founded High Point Hospital we decided we would make provision for both open and closed-ward facilities in order to carry a patient through an illness regardless of the nature of his behavior and the stage of his affliction. By and large we have been able to do this. Our object has been to keep the same therapist available for the patient throughout his illness, which cannot be the case if the hospital facilities are inadequate and it becomes necessary to transfer a patient to another hospital when he becomes difficult to manage.

The atmosphere of such a hospital cannot be regulated by edict. It is determined by the quality and character of the personnel, their organization and proper integration into the individual departments, their training, their interest in the work they are doing, and the extent to which this interest can be maintained. Of extreme importance, too, is a high ratio of doctors, nurses and aides for patients, if intensive therapy is to be carried out successfully. In order to implement our program, for instance, we have one active psychiatrist for every five to six patients, and one nurse or attendant for 1.7 patients. This permits a minimum of 3 psychotherapeutic hours per week per patient, over and above a great deal of personal attention by the therapist, and a rather highly individualized management by the nursing personnel.

The medical staff, if—as is the case at our Hospital—it happens to be psychoanalytically oriented, must be intensely interested in its work, and enough stout of heart not to become pessimistic in the face of slow progress. The work of residents must be closely supervised, and conferences on their cases should be held regularly and frequently. (We have been fortunate indeed to have three trained analysts available both for the individual treatment of patients, as well as for the supervision of the residents' work.) Conferences must be held regularly to evaluate and re-evaluate the progress of patients and their program of management. In addition, clinical conferences with the nursing staff about individual patients must be held. We have also found it very helpful to conduct a modest psychiatric aide training program to raise the level of alertness of our attendants. The nurse and aide are thus integrated into the therapeutic team.

We have found it extremely valuable to assign a significant role to the Directress of Nursing. She is required to participate in the psychiatric conferences so that she may convey the sense of them to her staff for proper handling of individual patients, and to convey to patients the rationale of rules and regulations as they are made or changed to meet changing requirements. Properly trained and interested, such a person can be a really constructive force in a psychotherapeutic hospital.

With the kind of atmosphere and organization I have outlined, it becomes possible to treat a variety of patients psychotherapeutically under the same roof. The acute and chronic schizophrenic, the depressive, mildly suicidal patient, as well as a carefully selected case of alcoholism or drug addiction may be treated for varying lengths of time.

A psychotherapeutic hospital can treat patients who would otherwise in private practice offer a poor prognosis. It includes a group of patients who are not functioning adequately, and are too sick to participate in analytic treatment on an ambulatory basis. They are the patients who may become worse soon after therapy is started. They cannot examine their own pathological processes, or when they do verbalize freely, they become hopelessly immersed in their own pathology and become increasingly disorganized.

Being in a hospital, however, is not of itself curative for such patients, although their disorganization may be stemmed. While in the hospital, the patient may secure a temporary remission and be subject to subsequent decompensations; or he may "get along" as a chronic hospital patient. The psychotherapeutic hospital, on the other hand, makes possible a dynamically oriented therapy that can result in durable improvement. Such a hospital offers specific conditions which make up for the deficiencies of the office setting for treatment of these patients.

The psychotherapeutic hospital is also helpful because everything the patient does and most of his reactions can be known to the therapist. The therapist does not have to depend on the patient to tell them to him. This reduces some of the handicaps we have in office practice. The therapist, who is able to see the patient for only one hour three to five times a week, knows very little of what goes on the rest of the time, except as the patient tells him of it. The very sick patient tells rather little, is too defensive, or unaware of much that is important. Furthermore, he may become disorganized when he feels compelled to tell too freely what is going on inside of him. In a hospital, the therapist, by himself, and through the assistance of a trained aide and nursing staff, can make up for this deficiency through a 24-hour observation of the patient. He can then take into account what he knows of the patient's dynamics, and judiciously introduce his observations in therapy for exploration. In this way the therapist can structure what is explored and analyzed in the treatment.

The patient who is no longer functioning adequately cannot rely on himself. Just as he cannot be depended upon to cooperate in therapy in the way a neurotic does, he cannot be depended upon to act in a responsible manner in his everyday life. His life and his behavior have to be supervised. In the hospital he is supervised and limits are put on his freedom of movement because his activity tends to be self-defeating, as well as hurtful to others. The supervision and limitations aid him in defining reality, as well as maintaining the integrity of his personality. However, this in itself is never curative, because it always promotes in these patients an active conflict between their dependency needs and their aggressive reactions against authority.

In the analytic hospital this basic conflict can be analyzed and insight achieved. The supervision and limitations then have a lasting value. We have found that one of the significant areas of exploration is the area of conflict emanating from the patient's reaction to authority and his need for guidance and help. An analytic approach to this conflict is made easier when the patient is removed from the authority represented by parents, marital partners, employers, and the like. The patient often sees these people only as negative influences, and often he is correct. He can, however, more readily appreciate the fact that hospital supervision is in his own interest because both authority as well as therapeutic intervention are employed judiciously to promote insight.

Once a patient's dynamics are known to an analyst working in a hospital setting, the analyst can employ a trained aide and the nursing staff, in a flexible manner, to provide the patient with the therapy he needs at any given time. When firmness is needed, firmness can be used, when permissiveness is needed, permissiveness can be applied. Similarly, the type of aide assigned to a patient, the amount of attention he receives, as well as its concentration at any time, can be controlled. When necessary, the patient may be left to his own devices, too, and a study made of the effect.

Under such circumstances the patient is not compelled to fight his environment. Rather, he finds that he is being encouraged to participate in it at his own pace, while the pathologic devices he had employed to evade society are not crushed, but, rather patiently examined, so that in time he may discard them voluntarily. The hospital society aims to help the patient realize mental health by becoming a rationally participating member of it.

We have found that there is a general tendency to avoid hospitalization as long as possible, not merely because of the expense involved, but more often because of the "stigma" attached to the idea and the traumatic effect on the patient that is feared. As a consequence, the patient may get to the hospital in pretty bad condition and require a more prolonged stay than may have been necessary. Our experience has shown that hospitalization need not at all be a traumatic experience, that with encouragement many patients will seek hospitalization quite voluntarily, and that the earlier the hospitalization, the better the outlook. Earlier hospitalization for patients may be achieved by disabusing both the patient and relatives, and perhaps ourselves, of unfounded anxieties about hospital care.

One's reluctance to hospitalize the psychotic patient is most marked, of course, when the patient's functioning is relatively unimpaired, and when he clashes little with others in society. Yet it is a fact that some of these people are more profoundly sick than the acutely disturbed patient, and that, as a rule, they offer a more guarded prognosis. The biggest problems are presented by patients who quietly go about their business, and sometimes are in treatment, and more often, are not. They don't fit into the commonly accepted indications for hospitalization until they become acutely disturbed and deluded, are overcome by depression or anxiety, or when they become a threat to themselves or to society. Prolonged care is then inevitable.

This type of patient requires early ambulatory treatment and early hospitalization. It would seem necessary to work out the earliest indications for hospitalization, particularly when, in the institution selected, psychotherapy is available.

There is little choice, and the situation is quite obvious, when the patient has gotten completely out of hand. Proper hospitalization should, however, be a matter of deliberation and premeditated choice rather than that of urgent necessity.

The hospital devoted to psychotherapy can be of real help to the practicing psychotherapist who often will struggle on with a very slow-moving, difficult, and even regressing patient for fear that the alternative is an unpleasant and unproductive hospitalization. Such an institution can pursue the course the therapist has been following, and do it in a controlled, planned atmosphere which offers a good chance of success. Once the patient has improved sufficiently—having worked out, perhaps, some transference problems—he may gradually renew his contact with his former therapist. We have seen this work out quite well.

There are times when a psychotherapist believes that he should no longer treat a particular patient, and yet does not feel free to broach the subject to the patient for fear that he will react to it badly, or even become acutely psychotic, before an adjustment to another private therapist has been made. In such an instance, hospitalization can help by serving as a bridge to another therapist. Under the more controlled conditions, the patient can make progress with the hospital therapist, and then, after leaving the hospital, he may make an easier change to another therapist.

It is unfortunate that when a patient is at his worst and has to be hospitalized, he is—as a rule—treated by a resident in training. This is one reason why a skilled private therapist hesitates to hospitalize a patient he has been treating. We have been meeting this problem at High Point not merely by closely supervising our advanced residents, but by having an attending staff of psychoanalysts at our service who actively treat about 30 per cent of our patients.

We believe that one of our very significant functions is to introduce to the patient the meaning and importance of psychotherapy. Frequently a patient will have his first experience with psychotherapy in a hospital devoted to this form of treatment. He has become acutely upset, seen a psychiatrist once, and been referred for hospitalization. Treated as outlined above, he has a relatively productive experience with a psychotherapist for the first time in his life, and may then voluntarily undertake psychotherapy after leaving the hospital.

Should the patient become psychotic during private treatment, a successful hospitalization with psychotherapy will keep him from losing his faith in it, and save him for a future ambulatory psychotherapy.

The hospital devoted to psychotherapy will naturally relegate the physiological therapies to their proper place. It is a fact today that in mental hospitals patients either soon receive shock treatments or are subjected to a custodial type of program which permits the self-limiting aspects of the psychotic attack to come to bear. The psychotherapeutic program can resist the pressure for shock treatment, and certainly rule out a merely custodial program. There are times, however, when shock treatment must be used as a life-saving measure, or for other well-considered reasons. No matter what the purpose, however, shock treatment should never be used as therapy per se, but adjunctive to the psychotherapeutic regimen itself.

I do believe, though, that we do not as yet know enough about the shock therapies to use them indiscriminately. I would guess that their true function, and value, if any, will be ultimately discovered only when the patient is, at the same time, subjected to intensive psychiatric study.

There are many patients for whom shock treatment is contraindicated for physical reasons. The hospital devoted to psychotherapy can save these patients from a custodial-type of hospitalization and an otherwise poor prognosis, and save those for whom shock treatment might be psychologically harmful.

The hospital devoted to psychotherapy has some specific problems. Its personnel must be quite carefully selected and be above average in intelligence and emotional stability. It is by no means an easy matter to secure such personnel. A major problem is to keep costs of operation within bounds so that the rates may remain within reason. Under any circumstances, the fees for such a program must be relatively high, if it is to live up to its standards. The pressure of relatives (and sometimes of psychiatrists) for a "quick cure" and an as-short-as-possible hospitalization manifests itself in demands for the use of shock treatment. It is sometimes quite a problem to convince the relatives that the psychotherapeutic procedure is surer, and only apparently slower. It is not easy to convince them, particularly if it is the patient's first hospitalization, that there are no miracle cures, and that the long-view, well-planned program is the best.

The major problem, however, for psychotherapy in a mental hospital stems from the relative lack of experience psychiatry has had with the operation of hospitals devoted to psychotherapy. There are only a handful of such hospitals in the country at present, and none of them has operated as such for too long. In psychiatry there is no weight of tradition to support them, let alone weight of public opinion. I do have the impression, however, that pioneering work has yet to be done in this area, and that there is much room for research not merely as to techniques of therapy, but also, importantly, as to the nature of hospital organization and administration.

A hospital devoted to psychotherapy should make a major effort to study, as well as treat, schizophrenia which—without being unduly dramatic—may be considered a scourge of modern civilization. Success in this area may lift the pall of pessimism which surrounds the treatment of this illness. We do achieve positive results with psychotherapy in a hospital setting and may, therefore, feel more optimistic about its treatment in practice.

So far, the bulk of institutions are geared to handle patients with more advanced symptomatology. It is difficult to say whether most hospitals are as they are because of the public's reluctance to hospitalize patients in the earlier stages of illness, and thus are forced to adopt the pattern of care for the more advanced cases, or whether the public is reluctant to seek hospital care because of the way existing mental institutions are organized. Whatever the case, it would seem in order to establish criteria for the proper kind of administrative and therapeutic atmosphere essential to the treatment of early schizophrenia.

There are just a few further matters I should like to touch upon. Some of you know that it was but a mere two years ago that I uprooted myself from a full psychoanalytic practice to found and organize High Point Hospital. This was the fruition of an idea some ten years old at the time. Now I would like to make known the fact—or confess—for the first time in public, that I did not know what I was getting myself into.

There is quite a difference between the ideal and the reality, between the idea and its fulfillment. When in private practice, I envisioned the manner in which I believed a hospitalized patient should be treated. In some respects it is still a vision, because of the many practical factors over which it is most difficult to exercise control. Yet these factors influence psychotherapeutic techniques and results. However, this gap between ideal and reality probably exists mainly because relatively little is known about the true nature of the psychotic process, and the kind of hospital society in which it can be understood and cured.

There were times during the reading of this paper when I may have sounded quite positive in my assertions. If I have, it was not with intention, for I could hardly pretend that a short two years of such experience would entitle me to be any more than tentative. It is more in the spirit of inquiry and to invite your comments that the paper is presented. The kind of experience we have had the past two years does not fall to—or befall—many psychiatrists, and I thought we should share what we have profited from it with you. And at the same time I wish to expose our shortcomings to your criticism.

We may conclude that there is room for the hospital devoted to psychotherapy, and that psychotherapy used with conviction has a very useful function in it. Such a hospital may serve many significant purposes, both for the patient, and for the referring psychiatrist. Its essential purpose is to furnish insight of a curative nature in a controlled atmosphere which can both tolerate the patient's unhealthy behavior, and fortify him gradually as he masters newly-developing healthy behavior.

As a rule the mental institution is considered a place to which one dreads sending a patient, and from which it is felt he must depart at the earliest possible moment, because there are unhealthy people in it. This seems to be the rule, even though it was among the normal people that the patient became sick, and among the ill ones that he regained his balance.

The properly organized psychotherapeutic hospital, however, should be regarded as a place where basic gains are made, and solidified, and from which a patient may emerge, not merely as well as ever, but healthier than ever. As such it need neither be dreaded nor fled. It is sad and disheartening to witness patients enter the hospital after they have been sick for several years only to leave long before they have obtained the fullest benefit from hospitalization. Basically, the soundness of a remission rather than the quickness of it should determine the length of hospitalization.

The hospital devoted to psychotherapy should offer an atmosphere—the exact kind yet to be determined—which will hold patients to it until they are sufficiently improved to fend for themselves. Psychotherapy should demonstrate its own value to the patient so that he continues it voluntarily. Finally, such hospitalization should be a living experience for the patient from which he can derive long-lasting, if not permanent, benefits which will enhance his ability to live more rationally, happily, and productively.

2

Adjunctive Shock Treatment in an Intensive Psychotherapeutic Program: Psychodynamic and Other Considerations

ALEXANDER GRALNICK, M.D.

SINCE THE INTRODUCTION of shock treatment many thousands of articles have been written on the subject. They have stemmed from the devoted labors of many workers in the field of psychiatry. It is not to their discredit that, nevertheless, its value is a matter of controversy. In a generation we have witnessed the introduction of insulin, metrazol, sulphur-in-oil, carbon dioxide and electro-shock therapy administered in a variety of ways, and with varying results. In more recent years we have entered upon the era of the tranquilizing agents, reputed and shown to be as, if not more, effective than the other modalities. We have experienced waves of enthusiasm and have been swept with the full-tide of optimism, only to be tugged by the ebb back to the reality of the tremendous task mental illness yet presents us. For the moment, we are riding the crest of the new chemicals, and the use of the shock modalities threatens to be washed into the discard.

Innumerable factors account for such a train of events in the history of psychiatry. This paper, however, neither would

---

Reprinted from *Congress Report of the II International Congress for Psychiatry,* Zurich (Switzerland) September 1957, Vol. II, pp. 380-386.

deal with them, nor attempt to put an end to the existing controversy. The speaker recognizes that the proponents of psychotherapy have added fuel to the fire, in many instances extolling the virtues of their method and condemning the use of organic procedures. Even within their own camp, sharp differences about techniques have existed. This paper would certainly not dare to calm these troubled waters, nor would it wish to introduce further controversy.

Fifteen minutes is indeed a short time in which to kaleidoscope some fifteen years of training and experience in the use of both the physiologic and psychotherapeutic procedures. It may perhaps be best accomplished by describing our experience in constructing and conducting our programme at High Point Hospital. In starting an institution devoted to psychoanalytically oriented psychotherapy many questions, naturally, arose. Should we be purists and exclude the shock therapies? How would this be viewed by the greater number of psychiatrists we were intending to serve? Would we serve a better purpose as psychotherapeutic purists? Could we? Would this be in the best scientific tradition? In introducing both modalities would we deny ourselves the chance to sift the wheat from the chaff? Which course would offer our patients the better programme? Could we disregard the worthy clinical reports from both camps? Would the presence of both modalities be a disservice one to the other? Could we exist if devoted exclusively to one form of therapy?

Time yielded the answers. Practical and clinical experience taught us the way. The psychiatrists who called upon us wished that we have both shock and psychotherapy available for their patients. While they did not wish us devoted exclusively to shock treatment, neither did they wish us solely to use psychotherapy. This held true regardless of the general approach of the psychiatrist—whether he held to an organic or functional orientation, and whether orthodox or unorthodox in his psychoanalytic derivation.

Clinical experience showed too that only a highly selected

group could be treated with psychotherapy exclusively. To pursue any such course would mean denying the benefit of our ability to many patients. It meant that any error in the selection of a patient who proved unmanageable or refractory to psychotherapy alone would mean his transfer to another institution with the consequent trauma entailed. Similarly, if devoted exclusively to shock therapy, it meant that the patient who failed to respond would suffer the trauma of transfer elsewhere away from his therapist.

In our initial stages we were devoted almost exclusively to psychotherapy. However, the experiences and considerations described dictated our course. As we introduced the freer use of shock treatment other questions and considerations came to the fore. What would be the effect on the patients as a group? Would individual patients lose confidence in us as psychotherapists or would they lose faith in psychotherapy itself? Would patients resist psychotherapy, if shock treatment was readily available and seemed an easier way to improve? Would the use of shock treatment interfere with the effectiveness of psychotherapy as some psychiatrists believed? Would the "miraculous" cure with shock treatment tend to shorten hospitalization so that patients would lose the opportunity for insight-therapy, and thereby be more easily a victim of relapse? What effect would there be on the relatives of patients?

These were but some questions which began to arise.

The manner and method of using shock treatment was much less of a problem. From my previous experience I believed that psychotherapeutic factors were at play in the results achieved with shock treatment. While they had never been "proven" scientifically, I had little question of it. My experience with shock treatment at Central Islip State Hospital had already alerted me to feel that it might be merely adjunctive to psychotherapy.

Our institution certainly offered an opportunity to test this thinking. While there was much to be said for each side, no one had a proven case, nor did it seem important that there be one. Clinical experience indicated that important physical and psychological forces were at work. What better atmosphere could there be to study them than one which would use both objectively as the clinical condition of the patient warranted. A rich opportunity to study the psychotherapeutic aspects of shock treatment would seem to exist where a patient was intensively treated and studied under psychotherapy. His emotional and psychological reactions to shock treatment, whether given or not, could become known as under no other conditions of study. This knowledge could only enhance our knowledge of psychodynamics, and clarify the psychological factors which would seem to contribute to the beneficial results following the administration of shock treatment. Such knowledge would be useful to our understanding of mental illness, without having to be placed in the service of proving its functional or organic etiology.

Thus, with these considerations in mind, we gradually but definitely introduced the use of shock treatment. All of our patients, however, remained exposed to an intensive program of psychotherapy. Essentially we are an institution maintaining a ratio of one active therapist for each five patients, each of whom receives three to five hours of psychotherapy per week. In addition each of the forty patients receives a great deal of individualized attention from the medical staff. The greatest number of patients enter and stay voluntarily for periods ranging up to several years. No custodial care is given, and an atmosphere of therapeutic optimism prevails.

If any principle guided us from the start it was that the patient selected for shock treatment would receive it only as his clinical condition dictated. In other words, there would neither be a fixed number of treatments nor a fixed pattern of administration. It was, of course, recognized that no experimental design was being constructed. However, it was believed that the situation was rather unique, and that after several years of such a pattern we would learn something, make observations worth transmitting to the profession and collect data which could be studied. It was not planned that the findings and observations have strict scientific validity, or give conviction to any greater extent than any clinical study is entitled.

As the use of shock treatment became integrated into our program, one of the first things we noted was a favorable psychological effect upon ourselves. We felt less handicapped. This was true in various circumstances, including the following:

1. Seriously suicidal patients, and those otherwise unmanageable.

2. Acutely disturbed states during the course of psychotherapy and stages of impasse when every known therapeutic technique proved useless.

3. In the involutional psychoses which did not respond to psychotherapy, or were associated with threatening physical states or accompanied by financial or other practical considerations which limited extended hospitalization. Under such circumstances shock treatment began to prove itself an essential adjunct that helped us overcome a sense of powerlessness in the face of uncontrollable conditions. Our psychotherapeutic efforts were thereby enhanced.

It became our responsibility, however, to refine our observations so that shock treatment was not given indiscriminately, but at the proper time and to the properly selected patient. We had to feel that it was given without prejudice and without limiting the patient's opportunity to profit from psychotherapy. It behooved us to explore the psychological effects of merely considering the desirability, let alone the actual administration of shock treatment.

The latter necessity required us to be particularly sensitive to the reactions of the individual patient as well as the patients as a group. This was especially true because the patients were a small and intimate group of people who knew much of what was going on about them and established close ties among themselves. The effect of shock treatment was readily apparent to most of the patients.

With time the patients accepted shock treatment as an additional facet of the armamentarium of the medical staff, without prejudice to the psychotherapeutic arm of the program. The latter was accepted as essential, everyday custom, whether or not shock was also being used in any individual case.

The patients showed no loss of faith in the medical staff. Some anticipated shock treatment with dread, whether the staff contemplated it for the patient or not, whereas others welcomed it as a source of hope should their efforts at insight-therapy fail. Its effect on other patients was noted with interest. On the basis of such observation a patient might actually ask for shock treatment, though sometimes only to avoid the anxiety of working out a problem, or to avoid the extended hospitalization a fellow-patient on psychotherapy might be having. Some patients would consider themselves "sicker" if shock treatment were used, but by the same token some considered the need for extended psychotherapy as a serious sign, and would accept shock treatment to shorten hospitalization and thereby deny the gravity of their illness.

The close study of patients who receive shock treatment while undergoing intensive psychotherapy has led us to certain observations and dynamic formulations of interest. They are not related as necessarily explaining the beneficial effects of shock treatment. Nor does their exposition suggest they are universal.

On the basis of our Hospital experience, we believe that shock therapy may be considered a valuable adjunct to intensive psychotherapy. We do not find that it interferes with insight-therapy. Rather we have witnessed it to facilitate psychotherapy. While, as yet, we can not offer statistical "proof" for our belief, we feel that our clinical impression is amply supported by the nature of our experience and practice.

No matter what physiological procedure is ever used, a constant will always be the psychology of the human organism. This constant must always be significant in determining results and, therefore, given due weight. Psychodynamic factors are properly appreciated when studied in the person actually subjected to the physiologic procedure. However, neither physical nor psychological methods at present offer us a final understanding of the origins and cure for mental illness. At best they offer us a bit more understanding and perhaps, at this stage, we would do well to be content with that.

The field of medicine is yet biased in favor of the physical aspects of disease. Research is naturally, therefore, weighted in favor of the physiologic. Until this unhealthy balance is corrected in our research and treatment efforts there is little likelihood that "the answer" to mental illness will be found, either in terms of its origins or effective treatment.

It is safe to say that none of us is too satisfied with what has been accomplished to date. We appreciate that none of our vaunted discoveries has given us the lasting results we desire for our patients. It may be that "the answer" to mental illness may never be found, but this is a premise none of us would care to adopt. Accordingly, we must afford a two-pronged approach.

Complicated and occult as are the physiological mechanisms of the body, as complex and mysterious are the psychological. The latter must be understood equally well, however, if our knowledge of the former is to really help us. This would seem to be so because a psychological response is the inescapable accompaniment of any physical procedure.

Such thinking as this is the basis of our treatment program. We recognize it to have limitations and deficiencies. However, we believe that work done along similar lines, perhaps with a more comprehensive research design, will enhance our understanding of mental illness immeasurably.

Any study limited exclusively to either the physical or psychological will not be conclusive or scientific in the true sense of the word. It can only be repetitive and confirm us in what we already know. The adjunctive use of shock treatment in a psychoanalytically-oriented program of psychotherapy, however, produces effective results and enhances our understanding of the mentally ill. It has a rationale and effects the progress of patients. One form of treatment is helpful to the other.

We have seen patients who by their history would not at all be expected to respond to shock treatment given alone, and as it ordinarily is, show good improvement when the shock therapy is given at the proper time during intensive psychotherapy and in the presence of a good transference relationship. We recognize that at times the latter is not enough, and the aid of shock treatment is sorely needed. It is also true that the shock treatment may only be of temporary help even at such time, just as shock alone will often be of temporary help. These facts, however, do not minimize the significance of either.

The immediately foregoing statements are far from definitive, and perhaps may even be confusing. But this is neither the fault of the psychiatrist, nor that of psychiatry. Neither is it a reason for apology, defensiveness or particularly pessimism. These are the facts, and they shed clarity for those who are ready to accept them objectively and to maintain the enthusiasm necessary to attain the final truth. They may be distressing to those who seek simple and accustomed answers because they cannot accept our present impotence. Some may actually use such facts unwittingly to create confusion and pessimism. Doing so, however, can only be a disservice to psychiatry.

We know that a patient with a particular diagnosis, and certain symptoms, who has not been sick unduly long, will respond quite well to shock treatment. We know too that his improvement may be short-lived, and that a matched patient may not respond at all to similar treatment. We have made exhaustive studies of the symptoms and responses of such matched patients, and also of the treatment techniques used. However, their personalities, and their psychodynamics have not been similarly studied. The personality-structure and the psychology of the patient treated by shock may be as significant to the outcome as his symptom-picture. Patients with similar symptoms may have an entirely different psychology, and it is this fact which may account for dissimilar results.

A programme devoted to the depth study of patients who are simultaneously exposed to adjunctive shock treatment offers an opportunity to determine the part the patient's psychology plays in the end-results achieved. All that our experience to date has taught us in this regard cannot be related in so few minutes. However, a few comments may be illustrative.

When depression is a prominent symptom it is expected to respond to shock therapy. However, one patient with it may improve whereas another, who is otherwise much the same too, may not improve at all with an equal number of or more shock treatments. Close study shows each to be sick, and mainly depressed, for different psychological reasons. The first has never been able to depend on or trust people, and has become sick under circumstances which have destroyed his independence. He does not respond to psychotherapy because he cannot trust his therapist, depend on him or give him due credit for helpful insight. It is much easier for him to credit the shock machine because it still allows him his independence from people. The other patient has become depressed for entirely different reasons, and views shock treatment as the ultimate proof of his weakness and inadequacy. He feels humiliated that he has been unable to manage without a mechanical procedure. Its need is no source of ego-support to him. He experiences it as a defeat and degradation. Physiological changes cannot counterbalance these psychodynamic forces.

Patients may show significant improvement with psychotherapy but yet not enough to warrant their release. For various reasons, including the honest judgment that shock treatment will be of some aid, the physical procedure is employed. Under such circumstances patients will react differently. Some who improve will disregard the help the therapist has been and attribute all to the shock treatment alone. Others will minimise its significance, and believe they would have gotten well nevertheless, or maintain that it was really the psychotherapist who deserves all the credit.

We have observed that factors of an emotional and psychological nature operate both in ourselves and the patients when shock treatment is considered. The patient who is dependent and helpless may plead for relief of his symptoms during psychotherapy, particularly if he is anxious at the prospect of working through a severe problem. When a transference-countertransference situation exists, the therapist may fall prey to the patient's pleas, implicit or explicit, and decide to administer shock treatment. He may actually fear failing the patient without shock therapy, and the patient may have succeeded in making him feel this way. When alert to this the therapist may make use of these dynamics in working through the resistances to insight, whether the patient improves with the shock or not. If not alert to these factors, the psychotherapist loses an opportunity to aid the patient psychologically. In administering shock merely on the basis of clinical symptoms we limit our awareness of the patient's personality. If we look deeper we find that hidden factors determine our choice as much as do observable symptom-complexes.

It appears often that we are submitting to the patient's implicit demand that we accomplish something magical. Patients in psychotherapy tend to clothe their therapists with super-human qualities, and expect him to accomplish the miraculous, so that they will not be disappointed in him. If he has to feel omnipotent a therapist is prey to such a situation, in which case both his and the patient's overdetermined needs are satisfied. At best this is a superficial solution, and contributes only to an unstable result.

It is true that at times the psychodynamics may be well known to both but the patient is too sick to permit their analysis. In such event the shock therapy may succeed in improving symptoms through a repression of the disturbing elements. Again, something of only a superficial nature has been accomplished, but at least the preliminary effort at psychotherapy gives us choice in the matter. In the process a transference relationship is established, and this is helpful in furthering any progress which may be stimulated by the shock treatment. In fact, we believe that the preliminary psychotherapy, though apparently of no aid, has set the stage for the shock to be of help. We have seen many patients whose history would indicate completely negative effects with straight shock respond to it after a preliminary period of psychotherapy lasting several months. We have seen many patients admitted immediately after failing to respond to shock therapy given elsewhere, show substantial improvement when given further shock treatment preceded by a period of psychotherapy. Of course, too, we have seen such patients respond to psychotherapy without the necessity of having to resort to shock treatment at all.

Shock treatment is a major and shaking experience in the life of a patient. In a brief span of time it repeatedly renders him unconscious and faces him with the prospect of death. It is not an average or common type of experience, and offers the psychotherapist an opportunity to evoke positive feelings because of his role in guiding the patient through it. In fact, the period of treatment provokes a flood of emotions which are directed at and shared with the therapist who has already made a relationship with the patient during the preliminary psychotherapy. However, what has heretofore appeared a rather nebulous, and poorly defined contact now blossoms into a productive and fruitful relationship as the therapist guides, re-orients, supports both physically and emotionally, suggests, and interprets this as well as other major experiences in the life of the patient.

It is often said that shock treatment impairs the patient's ability to utilize psychotherapy. Although patients may not recall the content of a session while receiving concurrent shock, they experience an intensification of their relationship to the therapist. The affective bond to the psychotherapist is spared the fate of the ideational content of their time spent together. The patient remains aware that his therapist has shown him interest and rendered some help. As a result there is further, though unapparent, progress in the relationship.

Without fear of contradiction one may say that the chronic schizophrenic who responds in any favorable manner to shock treatment does so because of the effected physiological changes. The problem, however, is not done justice by permitting the matter to rest there without a thorough investigation of the obvious and subtle psychodynamic forces operating between the patient and those about him.

So long as we conceive of mental illness as either physical or functional in nature, we must think of a modality as helping in terms of this belief. If shock treatment is of aid, the physiological changes produced by it must be thought the cause of such improvement, and by like token such a finding must be taken to be the proof of the physical origin of the illness. If psychotherapy is remedial the non-physiologic nature of this modality must be thought the cause of it, and this finding taken to be the proof of the functional origin of the disease. The pursuit of either approach without serious regard to the other, as has been the custom to date, will likely tell us little more basically than we already know. We will follow a will-o'-the-wisp. The writer is not prepared to say more than concerted effort must be made to discover a different approach to the understanding and treatment of mental illness.

3

Inpatient Psychoanalytic Psychotherapy of Schizophrenia: Problem Areas and Perspectives

ALEXANDER GRALNICK, M.D.

IN 1904 FREUD[1] SAID, "One should limit one's choice of patients to those who possess a normal mental condition. Psychoses are not suitable for psychoanalysis, at least not for the method as it has been practiced up to the present." However, he did add in the same article, "I do not regard it as by any means impossible that by suitable changes in the analytic method we may succeed in advancing beyond these hindrances, and so be able to initiate a psychotherapy of the psychoses."

However, in 1903 Freud[2] again cautioned that the psychoanalyst who selects a schizophrenic for treatment "has committed a practical error; he has occasioned useless expense and discredited his method of treatment; he cannot fulfill his promise of cure if the patient is suffering from paraphrenia (schizophrenia)." I believe that Freud's position never changed from this, though it is fair to say that numbers of the patients he described under different diagnoses would be considered cases of schizophrenia by most of us today. Again in 1914, in his paper "On Narcissism" Freud[3] said that as a consequence of having withdrawn his libido from

Presented at the Academy of Psychoanalysis, Philadelphia, April, 1959. Reprinted, by permission, from Science and Psychoanalysis, Vol. III *Psychoanalysis and Human Values,* edited by Jules H. Masserman, M.D. pp. 286-302. New York, Grune & Stratton, Inc., 1960.

persons and things in the outer world without replacing them by others in his fantasy, the schizophrenic is "inaccessible to the influence of psychoanalysis and cannot be cured by our endeavors."

Admittedly, the treatment of the schizophrenic is difficult and leaves our best efforts frequently unrewarded. The nature of such experience in its own right is enough to discourage an analyst. However, it is likely that Freud's beliefs have had a marked influence in promoting pessimism on a theoretical basis and discouraging disagreement with him on a clinical level. Fortunately, despite his proscriptions, some investigators have maintained the belief that the schizophrenic's withdrawal is by no means a complete one, and that despite a narcissistic regression some relatedness to other people continues to exist. Other students of the subject, considering that all human manifestations are meaningful—as did undoubtedly Freud—successfully studied the schizophrenic's mental and behavioral processes as comprehensible communications. In pointing this out Fromm-Reichmann indicated her belief that it was not the obscurity of the schizophrenic's communication "that constituted an obstacle to psychoanalytic psychotherapy with schizophrenics," and that "the reluctance to apply psychoanalytic knowledge and technique to the psychoses stems from Freud's paper on narcissisms,"[4] quoted above. In all fairness to Freud, however, it should be said that he proscribed "psychoanalysis," not "psychoanalytic psychotherapy," and believed that a transference relationship, as he described it, could not be profitably established with the schizophrenic.

Encouraged by Sullivan's teaching that interpersonal relatedness exists throughout all developmental periods and by the writings of others who also tended to revise Freud's concept, Fromm-Reichmann did her brilliant work with schizophrenics at Chestnut Lodge. It is fair to say that many of those who today work psychoanalytically with schizophrenics have been stimulated to do so by her belief that these patients are fit subjects for the psychoanalyst's techniques. However, it would be a mistake to think that the matter of the selection of the schizophrenic for psychoanalytic treatment is not a serious problem area yet begging for resolution. So long as doubts exist, so long will therapists be discouraged from serious efforts, and the work of those brave enough to explore this area will be regarded with question.

A second serious problem area in psychoanalysis concerns itself with determining and establishing the proper therapist-patient relationship. Starting with the declaration that the power of suggestion is implicit in the doctor-patient relationship, Freud tells us that "scientific psychotherapy" dictates that we "seek to control this factor, use it with a purpose, and direct and strengthen it." Against the possibility that anyone might think that by this he meant the analyst should actively exert personal influence over his patient, Freud, in 1912 said:

> The loosening of the transference is made more difficult by too intimate an attitude on the part of the doctor, so that a doubtful gain in the beginning is more than cancelled in the end. Therefore, I do not hesitate to condemn this kind of technique as incorrect. The physician should be impenetrable to the patient, and like a mirror, reflect nothing but what is shown to him. In practice, it is true, one cannot object to a psychotherapist combining a certain amount of analysis with some suggestive treatment in order to achieve a perceptible result in a shorter time—as is necessary, for instance, in institutions; but one may demand that he himself should be in no doubt about what he is doing and should know that his method is not that of true psychoanalysis.[5]

In 1913 Freud tells us "The first aim of the treatment consists in attaching him [the patient] to the treatment and to the person of the physician."[2] By this, I take it, he means establishing the transference relationship. While this suggests that Freud indicated that the analyst take an active role vis-a-vis the patient, I think it is fair to say that basically, as indicated above, he proscribed anything faintly resembling the interpersonal relationhip so actively sought and explored by the followers of the Sullivanian school. I say this despite an occasional statement by Freud suggesting he favored an active role in the more modern sense. For instance, he says at one time, "Does the uncovering of resistances automatically overcome them? Certainly not always. Our hope is to achieve this by exploiting the patient's transference so as to induce him to adopt the therapist's conviction of the inexpediency of the repressive processes established in childhood, and of the impossibility of conducting life on the pleasure principle."[6]

In 1919, Freud predicted that "Analysis will proceed in a direction described by Ferenczi as 'activity' on the part of the analyst,"[6] activity which puts the patient "into a mental situation most favorable to a solution of the conflict." As though to justify or rationalize this, Freud adds, "After all what the patient can achieve depends partly on a number of external circumstances which converge in their influence upon him."

Basically, however, Freud remained committed to a role of distance and aloofness from his patient. This is summed up in the following statement:

> Analytic treatment should be carried through, as far as is possible, under privation—in a state of abstinence. We must see to it that the patient's sufferings do not prematurely come to an end. Substitutive gratifications must be opposed, especially when sought in the treatment situation itself—in the transference relationship—when the patient tries to compensate himself through this means for all the other privations laid upon him—as far as his relations with the physician are concerned, the patient must have unfulfilled wishes in abundance. It is expedient to deny him precisely those satisfactions which he desires most intensely, and expresses most importunately.[6]

Some analysts, however, refused either to desert these patients or to deny them the benefit of their skills. Among these was Fromm-Reichmann. As already indicated, she believed that the schizophrenic maintained at least some ability to establish a workable transference relationship, and that his communications could be understood if analysts would but try to comprehend him and alter their techniques accordingly. She started with the belief that very early frustrations had so traumatized him that the schizophrenic became distrustful and drew into himself and away from reality, but at the same time maintained some awareness of his loneliness and longing for human contact. She says, "Certain groups of neurotics have to learn by the immediate experience of analytic treatment how to accept the denials life has in store for each of us. The schizophrenic has above all to be cured of the wounds and frustrations of his life before we can expect him to recover."[7] In keeping with this belief she gave the utmost of herself in sympathy and attempts at understanding to the schizophrenic.

Fromm-Reichmann had a warmth for the schizophrenic, particularly in the earlier years of her work with them, which cannot be conveyed by words. Those of us here who had the good fortune to hear her will know what I mean. Edith Weigert is perhaps the only person I know today who conveys in her spoken words this quality I am trying to describe. One gains the impression that Fromm-Reichmann gave much of herself and worked hard to establish the relationship of which she felt the patient capable. It was as though she would win the patient away from his retreat and heal his wounds by the very strength of her will, the depth of her desire to aid him and the warmth of her personality. She says, "There will remain long stretches on every schizophrenic's lonely road over which the analyst cannot accompany him, that is, not understand him. It is certainly not an intellectual comprehension of the schizophrenic but the sympathetic understanding and skillful handling of the patient's and physician's mutual relationship that are the decisive therapeutic factors."[7] Her compassion for the suffering schizophrenic is so evident here, as elsewhere in her earlier papers. Where she failed she blamed herself but not the patient. She says, "If the schizophrenic's reactions are more stormy and seemingly more unpredictable than those of the psychoneurotic, I believe it to be due to the inevitable errors in the analyst's approach to the schizophrenic, of which he himself may be unaware, rather than to the unreliability of the patient's emotional response."[7] Further, she says, "the schizophrenic is capable of developing strong relationships of love and hatred towards his analyst. In addition I believe the schizophrenic develops transference reactions in the narrower sense which he can differentiate from the actual interpersonal relationship."[7]

I have quoted at length from both Freud and Fromm-Reichmann to indicate the marked contrast in their ideas about the nature of the patient-analyst relationship, and the workability of the transference relationship. Essentially, this contrast exists in our thinking today. At one pole is the reserved and aloof technician; at the other extreme is the sympathetic and active therapist engaged in a life and death struggle to win the patient to his side.

What is already a complex problem becomes doubly so when we find that few are ready to agree on any definition of "classical technique" (Mohr[8]). Loewenstein says, "I do not know any foolproof definition of classical psychoanalysis."[9] Attempts are now made to draw the distinction between "variations," "modifications" and "deviations" from classical technique. How desperate or confused may some of us yet become? As we increasingly accept the fact that technique must be tailored to the patient's needs, and that he after all is our greatest variable, we will have to settle the conflict between our allegiance to our teachings and our responsibility to the clinical needs of patients.

In discussing method, Freud stated, in 1912, "This technique has proved to be the only method suited to my individuality."[5] Since the therapist's personality is so significant to successful treatment—and, I would guess, particularly so for the schizophrenic—certain questions would seem logical. Should most analysts give up the treatment of schizophrenia? Shall we change our personalities, or our general approach to the disease? Can we do so without fear that we are no longer "analysts"?

In a variety of ways Freud indicates that psychoanalytic technique is directed toward unearthing unconscious material in the face of the patient's resistance to this process as well as to his own recovery. The details of his method are sufficiently known not to need accounting now, and his personal approach to his patient has already been indicated. It is to Freud's credit that he anticipated improvements in technique by expressing "the hope that advances in the experience of psychoanalysts will soon lead to agreement upon the most expedient techniques"[5] for treatment. He did not at all believe that he had said the last word.

Freud's handling of the transference relationship has already been indicated. The fulcrum of the analytic work was the replacement of the ordinary neurosis by a transference neurosis of which the patient was then cured. Since the schizophrenic was not capable of establishing a transference relationship, no psychoanalytic techniques worthy of the name could be applied to him.

Fromm-Reichmann's early techniques relative to the doctor-patient relationship have already been indicated. With the passage of years she modified her approach. One can only guess that this was the result not merely of her mounting experience but also of developing changes in her own personality. The person who works intensively with schizophrenics is perhaps subject to such changes more readily than another. She indicates that her original "permissive, accepting" attitudes, strongly colored, I would guess, by her sensitive and strong sympathy for the schizophrenic's sufferings, was addressed to the "rejected child" part of the patient, and insufficiently to the "grown-up person" he had been before regressing. The change in her approach is quite apparent to one who follows her papers. She says that the schizophrenic senses that he cannot be helped by one person offering him a type of acceptance otherwise not mutually obtainable in adult society. It is more likely that she herself sensed this and became more realistic in her treatment techniques and more demanding of the patient. Realism probably replaced kindly and perhaps overplayed sympathies and identification—a countertransference phenomenon. In 1948, she said the analyst should address himself "on the level of the patient's present chronological age,"[4] which, in my own estimation, means a recognition on her part that the patient has normal areas of reality recognition upon which a therapist can draw.

Fromm-Reichmann says, "The psychoanalyst now acts as a participant observer and enlists the patient to collaborate in gaining insight into the genesis and dynamics of his illness."[4] She says further, "Those elements of the schizophrenic's relationship with the psychoanalyst, the transference character of which is obvious, should be used for analytic clarification," but, "only those elements which are an expression of the real positive interrelatedness between patient and analyst need not be touched by the therapist. Sooner or later the articulate schizophrenic will take care of their discussion by himself." We see that she believed the schizophrenic to be capable not merely of a transference relationship, but also of elements of a rather healthy one.

In papers written in 1939 and 1943 Fromm-Reichmann[7,10] suggests modifications in classical technique for application to the treatment of in-patient schizophrenics. These modifications include (1) a conscious and active attempt by the therapist to win the patient's confidence; (2) permitting the patient to sit up, rather than using the couch; (3) the use of structured expressions, rather than free association; (4) the evaluation of nonverbal expressions; (5) the analyst's conscious effort to show the patient that he is trying to help; (6) the therapist's expression of concern and sympathetic understanding; and (7) the withholding of too much and too free interpretation.

These modifications in technique would seem so drastic as to make one wonder whether "psychoanalysis" is being used. Fromm-Reichmann raises this question, but states that Freud believed that any therapy which accepted his teachings about the unconscious, about transference and resistance, and about infantile sexuality might be called psychoanalysis.

The consideration of the proper patient-therapist relationship and of the techniques for treatment of the schizophrenic logically lead to another problem area—that dealing with the social structure of the institution itself. One's basic conception of the nature of schizophrenia will depend on his training and experience with the disease process. In turn, it will determine the nature of one's therapeutic relationship to the patient as well as the treatment techniques one will employ. Similarly, it will decide the nature of the hospital for the in-patient schizophrenic.

The character of many institutions treating schizophrenics[11] has been decided by the belief that they are hopeless and incapable of relating in a meaningful way. Such places will be custodial in nature or depend solely on physiologic procedures to render any help. Even a hospital believing in the functional origin of schizophrenia will have its social structure determined by the nature of its staff's training and experience with the disease, the personalities of its policy makers, and their conception of the character of schizophrenia. The pure classicist who believes the schizophrenic too regressed to relate profitably is not likely really to expect analytic therapy to be very effective, or to believe that the nature of the social relationships existing therein will be of great consequence in the ultimate scheme of things.

It is likely that if one were to take time he would find that the evolution in the character of our institutions has paralleled our evolving concepts of the nature of mental illness. Fromm-Reichmann indicates in her earlier articles that she handled patients "with as much acceptance, permissiveness, and as little rejection as could possibly be administered—nothing short of actually destructive or suicidal action was prohibited."[7,4,10] One may well imagine the nature of the social relationships within an institution under such conditions. The theory was that the patient had already been so traumatized and rejected that he could not tolerate any frustration. Fromm-Reichmann does not indicate anywhere in her writings to what extent the problems created within her institution by such an approach had to do with the ultimate change in her beliefs.

When Fromm-Reichmann addressed herself to the patient "on the level of the patient's present chronological age," the nature of her relationship to the patient changed. Undoubtedly the nature of all social relationships within her institution changed accordingly too. One gains the impression, however, that she still depended on the one-to-one relationship between her and the patient fundamentally to effect a positive result. Unfortunately, she does not indicate what effect this change in her approach had on the nature of the institution itself.

Many factors have probably lead to the recrudescence of the concept of the therapeutic community. One of them may very well be the changing approach to the potentialities of the schizophrenic. When one conceives of the schizophrenic as capable both of profiting from relationships and contributing to them he is on the way to thinking of the therapeutic community as the best atmosphere for the in-patient. It becomes our job then to consider the ingredients which make such a community most wholesome for the schizophrenic, for it is a social system which gives the patient responsibility to the group as well as privilege within it.[12-14] The patient must, therefore, learn how to function within it as he has had to do in his family unit—only this time with success.

What are the elements within the therapeutic milieu which may serve a therapeutic function? Can we define them? Can we so construct and control the nature of interpersonal activity within an institution as to make its various elements subject to study? Can we so organize an institution and its activities so that they will by their very quality have a therapeutic effect on the patient? If social relationships in society have been of a kind to traumatize and produce disease process, can we construct a set of human relationships in which the schizophrenic will be healed? These are big questions.

We know that certain elements of the therapist-patient relationship, aside from techniques of treatment, have a healing quality. We have been accustomed, however, to think of these as inherent only in the one-to-one relationship of patient and analyst. Might they be transposed and reproduced in a group setting so as to have a similar effect on the patient, both consciously and unconsciously? The therapeutic relationship is designed to help through the furnishing of insight in the face of resistance. Yet insight and growth are an everyday accompaniment of life, apart from the therapeutic relationship. People have "spontaneous remissions" under certain conditions of life outside of a hospital, as well as within institutions otherwise bereft of every visible reason for any such thing happening. We are aware, too, that certain patients fail to respond despite very thoroughgoing insights. This is true to such an extent sometimes as to make one wonder whether "insight" is the entire answer.

May we give an environment some of the healing attributes of the doctor-patient relationship as we have developed it in psychoanalytic practice? Might we arrange things so as to permit the patient his compulsion to repeat with the freedom Freud suggested so that ultimately we, and he, might see the full depth of his pathogenic impulses? Freud suggests exploiting the transference relationship to induce the patient to adopt our conviction about the inexpediency of conducting life on the pleasure principle. Might we exploit the patient similarly through a special living arrangement which could be established in a hospital setting? Further, Freud's recommendation that the patient must have "unfulfilled wishes in abundance" and be denied "substitutive gratifications" might also find a place in an institution. Is it conceivable that Fromm-Reichmann's earlier ideas could be incorporated into a community setting? Under such conditions permissiveness would prevail, and all personnel would be expected to be sensitive, sympathetic and giving to the highest degree. The "rejected child" in the patient would be saved every trauma, frustration and rejection possible, and his every wish satisfied wherever humanly possible.

As a development of Fromm-Reichmann's later thinking we may conceive of the schizophrenic as having some rather strong ego qualities aside from his state of regression. We address ourselves "to the chronological age of the patient," and construct things to foster the more mature aspects of the patient's personality. We may then think of a milieu that takes these factors into consideration. We have been taking an approach of this nature at High Point Hospital. Under such conditions we may cushion the patient in certain areas, yet require things of him elsewhere which expose him to a certain degree of tolerable trauma and frustration from which experience he may learn about himself. At a determined stage of treatment a patient may be projected into certain group activities which place him under pressure and expose his problems relating to others. If timed properly, he may gather insight by himself, though the setting allows him to do so additionally with the aid of a therapist. At the proper time the patient is required to participate in the fulfillment of the needs of the society in which he is living and to learn of the problems he has in doing so. In this manner the difficulties he has in cooperating within a group, and submerging himself for the greater good are exposed. Overdetermined individualism and grandiosity are laid open for examination. In some ways a parallel is drawn with family living.

At the same time the patient has an opportunity to explore his problems in asserting his legitimate personal liberties. Exposure to parental and authority figures within the milieu is arranged with design in working group relationships, not merely in the one-to-one therapeutic situation. Simultaneously the patient may gather the strength that accrues from learning to work successfully with groups, and from being a respected member of a group.

In every way possible the hospital community is constructed to resemble the larger society. It is neither a retreat nor designed to relieve the patient of all pressures. It aims to exert pressures under relatively reasonable conditions, and thereby to furnish him an experience he has never quite had—an opportunity to grow and mature beyond a level he had ever achieved before in life. While the patient will tend to repeat his old patterns and at first see his experiences as no different from what he had known before entering the hospital, every effort of the therapeutic community is directed toward handling him differently enough that he may see it and mature as a result. This would be true particularly in relation to experiences with authority figures.

The analyst who is committed to the concept that effective change evolves only from the intimate one-to-one relationship of patient and doctor will take exception to the idea that the therapeutic community can be "therapeutic" in his sense of the word. In a like vein he will minimize the value of group therapy. His basic concept of the origins of mental disease will similarly differ from the psychiatrist who is oriented to thinking of mental illness as a reflection of family processes in a specific social context rather than a result of biological processes. The latter therapist will be more sympathetic to the value of the therapeutic community.

If schizophrenia is a distortion of normal human relationships and an outgrowth of biological drives in a conflicting social context, it would seem that a proper change in the patient's milieu would automatically be beneficial. If it is true that man's most precious asset is his fellow man and that without him he is both useless and devoid of human qualities, then the idea of specific social relationships as a therapeutic tool would seem to have validity. The "normal" community setting then would seem to promote change from sickness to health to the extent that it can encourage and enable the patient to take a rational, participating role.

Psychoanalysis may not be able much longer to point to its youth as a defense against not having reached greater agreement among its practitioners. It has a major responsibility here, particularly if it would lay claim to a right to treat an illness as malignant as schizophrenia. It would seem that we have come a long way in the past half century, and yet we are hardly as effective with the schizophrenic as we must eventually be. Is this a matter of our inadequate understanding, or of limiting concepts and hampering conditions? Are our techniques perhaps tradition-bound and we too narrow in the application of the knowledge we already have?

A modification of basic theory might have helped or been developed by Freud had he been more successful clinically with schizophrenics. Freud himself said, "As the transference neuroses have enabled us to trace the libidinal instinctual impulses, so dementia praecox and paranoia will give us insight into the psychology of the ego. Once more, in order to arrive at what is normal and apparently so simple, we shall have to study the pathological with its distortions and exaggerations."[3] In this manner he did encourage us to forge ahead. Should our ultimate findings suggest revisions in theory, we will more easily be able to make them if we are free in advance to see them.

Albert Einstein[15] said, "There are no eternal theories in science. It always happens that some of the facts predicted by a theory are disproved by experiment. Every theory has its period of gradual development and triumph." Basically the problem is that of determining the proper approach to the schizophrenic's treatment—not whether we are or are not doing "true psychoanalysis." Modifications in the therapy of schizophrenia may open the door to better ways of understanding and treating our more benign illnesses. As Freud said, "We have never been proud of the fullness and finality of our knowledge and capacity; as at the beginning, we are ready now to admit the incompleteness of our understanding, to learn new things and alter our methods in any way that yields better results."[6] May we ourselves do differently or be less brave?

REFERENCES

1. Freud, S.: On psychotherapy (1904). *In* Collected Papers. London, Hogarth Press, 1940, Vol. I, pp. 249-263.
2. ——: Further recommendations in the technique of psychoanalysis (1913). *In* Collected Papers. London, Hogarth Press, 1940, Vol. II, pp. 342-365.
3. ——: On narcissism (1914). *In* Collected Papers. London, Hogarth Press, 1940, Vol. IV, pp. 30-59.
4. Fromm-Reichmann, F.: Notes on the development of treatment of schizophrenics by psychoanalytic psychotherapy, Psychiatry *2*:263, 1948.
5. Freud, S.: Recommendations for physicians on the psychoanalytic method of treatment (19912). *In* Collected Papers. London, Hogarth Press, 1940, Vol. II, pp. 323-333.
6. ——: Turnings in the ways of psychoanalytic therapy (1919). *In* Collected Papers. London, Hogarth Press, 1940, Vol. II, pp. 392-402.
7. Fromm-Reichmann, F.: Transference problems in schizophrenics. Psychoanalyt. Quart. *8*:412, 1939.
8. Mohr, G. J.: Psychoanalysis: Some present-day assessments. *In* Masserman, J. H., Ed.: Psychoanalysis and Human Values. New York, Grune & Stratton, 1960.
9. Lowenstein, R. H.: Remarks on some variations in psychoanalytic technique. Internat. J. Psychoanalysis. *39*:202, 1958.
10. Fromm-Reichmann, F.: Psychoanalytic psychotherapy with psychotics. Psychiatry. *6*:277, 1943.
11. Gralnick, A., Schacht, M., and Kempster, S. W.: Psychotherapy in a private mental hospital. Am. J. Psychotherapy. *8*:312, 1954.
12. ——: Behavioral determinants in a therapeutic milieu. *In* Sarwer-Foner, G. J., Ed.: The Dynamics of Psychiatric Drug Therapy. Springfield, Ill., Charles C Thomas, 1959.
13. Cohen, R. A.: The hospital as a therapeutic instrument. Psychiatry. *21*:29, 1958.
14. Gralnick, A., and D'Ella, F.: Role of the patient in the therapeutic community: Patient-participation. Read at Southern Divisional Meeting of A.P.A., December, 1958. Submitted for publication.
15. Einstein, A., and Infield, L.: The Evolution of Physics. New York, Simon & Schuster, 1938.

patients lack the capacity for relatedness to other human beings. He cites also Fromm-Reichmann's contrary conviction (based upon experience) that the schizophrenic does possess this capacity and is thus a proper subject for psychoanalytic treatment. However, Gralnick acknowledges that the precise qualities that would serve to distinguish the analyzable psychotic from the unanalyzable one are not known and that the whole question is still arguable.

Gralnick next discusses the question of what constitutes a "proper" therapist-patient relationship and how it may be established. Again quoting Freud, he observes that this great originator felt that *suggestion* was a permissible adjunct to the psychotherapy of psychotics "in institutions," but that such treatment was definitely not psychoanalytic; for, after all was said and done, Freud regarded the analyst's proper role as basically one of aloofness from the patient. Fromm-Reichmann considered that schizophrenia is the result of severe trauma in early child-parent relations, such that the schizophrenic tends to distrust all people and to avoid human social reality. Nevertheless she observed that the schizophrenic is to some extent aware of his loneliness and that he yearns for human contact. She considered, therefore, that her role as therapist was to restore, through her own person, the schizophrenic's damaged faith in other human beings, and she devoted every resource of warmth she possessed to carrying out this endeavor. If she failed, she regarded the failure as her own rather than the patient's.

Gralnick finds that both these attitudes—Freud's recommended aloofness and Fromm-Reichmann's recommended warmth—exist among psychoanalysts today. He expresses the belief that the therapist's attitude of warmth or aloofness necessarily influences whether the patient remains aloof and inaccessible or tries to respond. But apart from this, Gralnick acknowledges that we are still in the dark as to the nature of a "proper" therapist-patient relationship.

The third question discussed by Gralnick is an outgrowth of the second. It concerns the matter of a "correct" psychoanalytic technique for dealing with the schizophrenic. Though few analysts agree on all the details of what constitutes a "classical" technique, many of them observe that the individual analyst may be confronted with the conflict presented, on the one hand, by his own need to be "loyal" to a given technique and, on the other, by the clinical needs of his patient: shall he be rigid or adjustable? Gralnick points out that the analytic therapist in whom such conflict arises must either change his own personality (how?) or refrain from treating schizophrenics. Fromm-Reichmann herself, with the passage of years, shifted her view of her role from that of the warm, all-giving, all-permissive mother to one in which she regarded her patient as being, in part or potentially, a grown-up person—not solely the rejected child. Gralnick astutely remarks that this shift was only partially the outcome of her mounting experiences with schizophrenics; it was also in part the result of "developing changes in her own personality." She says that her patients sensed that they could not ultimately be helped by a type of acceptance not otherwise "obtainable in adult society." Gralnick, again most astutely, notes that it is more likely that she herself sensed this and altered her role to one of more realistic demandingness toward her patients. He observes that a better orientation toward reality on her part had replaced what may have been countertransference in her earlier evaluation of her therapeutic role.

There were several occasions when I was privileged to open discussion of a paper of hers on schizophrenia. Regarding one of her earlier papers, I remarked that it appeared that she was approaching the therapy of schizophrenia in the spirit of the Spenserian device, "*Amor vincit omnia*" (love conquers all things); that, while genuine love can accomplish much, it is far from being, single-handedly, a panacea in the treatment of any ailment of the human personality. I was glad to observe, as her papers proceeded, the alteration in approach noted by Gralnick, and I remember that she was pleased with a comment of mine that her technique with schizophrenics was coming more and more to resemble the ordinary psychoanalytic technique.

Throughout this section of his paper Gralnick seems to have an uncommon degree of empathy with Fromm-Reichmann. While Fromm-Reichmann, according to published statements, thought she was utilizing psychoanalytic methods in her treatment of schizophrenics, Gralnick, level-headed here as elsewhere throughout the paper, reserves judgment as to whether Freud would have agreed with her.

The fourth, and final, question discussed relates to the ideal structure of a mental hospital attempting to deal psychotherapeutically with schizophrenics. The solution of this problem, as is the case with all the others, depends upon one's "theory" of schizophrenia. Those hospitals whose directors believe that schizophrenia is "incurable" will emphasize their custodial function and will utilize chemotherapy and electrotherapy with a view to rendering their schizophrenic patients more amenable to custodial efforts. For them the nature of the social structure of the hospital is inconsequential.

For other hospitals whose directors believe that schizophrenia has a psychogenesis, their social structure will be regarded as an important factor, and it is likely to undergo evolutionary change which parallels evolving concepts of the nature of schizophrenia. Fromm-Reichmann, for instance, thought that nothing short of obviously destructive or suicidal behavior should be prohibited to schizophrenic patients. She did not indicate in her writings whether, as her therapeutic attitude toward schizophrenic patients became more objective, she advocated corresponding changes in the social relationships within the hospital, but Gralnick conjectures that this was the case.

Resulting, however, from Fromm-Reichmann's more hopeful therapeutic attitude and the new experiences that emerged from this, the idea of the "therapeutic community" has now reappeared. Once it is accepted that the schizophrenic has certain potentialities which enable him both to respond to the society he finds in the hospital and to contribute something to it, this society becomes an important factor in his therapy, and hospital authorities have the tasks of determining what kind of social structure will be most beneficial therapeutically and of endeavoring to bring it into being. If we maintain the hypothesis that schizophrenia is the outcome, wholly or in part, of traumatic social relations, can we create a type of social structure in a mental hospital that will tend toward healing such damage? If such a structure could be created, could it in and of itself work therapeutically for the schizophrenic or would it have a beneficial effect only in conjunction with individual psychotherapy?

Gralnick raises these important questions, but he does not attempt to answer them. He sees clearly, however, the manner in which the patient's life within the hospital society might relate to two factors that Freud considered important in the psychoanalytic therapy of the individual: (1) the necessity of understanding that it is inexpedient to conduct one's life solely on the basis of the pleasure principle; (2) the necessity of imposing a degree of privation *(Versagung)* upon the patient undergoing psychoanalytic therapy. Genuine group living ("the therapeutic community") always entails the individual sacrifice of some pleasure whenever it would jeopardize the welfare of the group as a whole, and in some instances this principle necessarily involves a degree of privation for the individual. The therapeutic community can become a microcosm of the world at large and controlled in terms of the individual's needs and his tolerance of frustration, can produce new adjustments in the patient which will prepare him for better participation in extramural society when he leaves the hospital than was possible for him before entering it.

This thoughtful paper, based on a wide and concentrated experience, is an important contribution to our thinking on schizophrenia in general and, more particularly, to the problem of the management of the hospitalized schizophrenic.

4

Considerations in Evaluating the Results of Psychotherapy with 500 Inpatients

MAURICE H. GREENHILL, M.D.
ALEXANDER GRALNICK, M.D.
ROBERT H. DUNCAN, M.D.
RUSTU YEMEZ, M.D.
FARUK TURKER, M.D.

SEVERAL THINGS prompted us to make this study, some special aspects of which will be the subject of this paper. After about ten years of conducting a program emphasizing analytically oriented psychotherapy, a natural curiosity began to overcome us. A relatively small and simple program had evolved into a rather complex organism with many unforeseen ramifications. A few components had grown into many, and a small staff of people had flowered into a relatively large group, despite a fixed number of patients. An ordinary "institution" had become a complex society with its own peculiar system, standards, values, and laws. A place to which patients originally had been brought so that doctors could mainly render insight therapy had grown into a highly integrated social structure. Policies and treat-

Presented at the Second National Meeting of the Association for the Advancement of Psychotherapy, St. Louis, Mo., May 5, 1963. Reprinted from *American Journal of Psychotherapy,* Vol. XX, No. 1, pp. 58-68. January, 1966.

ment procedures seemed to change as did the type and characteristics of both patient-population and professional and nonprofessional staff. A meager group in a quiet rather empty building grew into a full organization in a hospital humming with activity.

What at first seemed simple, clear, and fully understandable had become complicated, replete with unknowns and somewhat incomprehensible. Nevertheless, therapeutic results which had been unacceptable earlier became increasingly good with time. Less travail brought forth better results even with more difficult patients. Greater awareness and therapeutic ability, however, were admixed with feelings of frustration which followed unaccountable failures. Growing clinical experience seemed to teach that more than the one-to-one psychotherapeutic relationship had become involved in the therapeutic results at our hospital. What was it, and how could we go about finding the significant factors? More than normal curiosity had now become involved.

It seemed natural to start with a large case study to see what it would show, and where it would lead us. True, we had many "clinical impressions" of what we had been accomplishing but they could hardly meet the requirements of objectivity. What type of case had we really been treating? How had we really been going about things? What were the results? Were they commensurate with the time, effort, and cost? Where were we falling down? How might our findings contrast with those of other private hospitals, and why? With public hospitals, and why? Were there any proven advantages to private hospital care as opposed to public care? If so, would such a study show what they were? Were the results better, or merely different because the treatment program was different? Could we ultimately find what program was better for a particular patient? These were some of the questions which occurred to us.

It seemed further that our findings would be of general if not particular interest. The profession seemed entitled to know more exactly what transpired in the proprietary, as well as public, hospital. Certainly it should prove enlightening from more than one vantage point.

The number of cases picked was determined with an eye to it being a representative and impressive sample that covered a good period of time as well. Our hospital had been started in 1951. Accordingly, 1956 was chosen as the first year to begin the study of case records. By that time the hospital was past its period of constant flux, and such a degree of stability and continuity had been achieved that policies and procedures had been committed to writing, although to this very day change remains a constant factor.

We had an additional reason for a retrospective study. What had psychotherapists, without specific fixed instruction, placed in their recordings? What had they emphasized? What had they omitted? Additionally, we hoped to learn what we would eventually want with uniformity in our records so that research could be done more easily. Our research team then entered the picture to determine what factors should be culled for study. The actual task thereafter of abstracting the data was done by two members of the clinical staff. At least 1,200 hours were spent in this phase of the study alone.

These introductory remarks indicate the inevitable growth of the complex structure needed to sustain a program emphasizing psychotherapy. They suggest the intricacy of factors which need to be considered in assessing its results.

It is not our present plan to emphasize statistics, but to indicate what must be pondered in the process of their gathering, and in evaluating the results of psychotherapy. The second section of the paper will deal with theoretical and methodologic considerations, and the third with certain variables at High Point Hospital which would seem to affect the results of psychotherapy.

THEORETICAL AND METHODOLOGIC CONSIDERATIONS

The evaluation of the results of psychotherapy is admittedly difficult. Most efforts to date in the assessment of results have dealt with the *intrinsic* factors relating to the one-to-one situation, that is, the doctor-patient relationship, transference and counter-transference aspects, interaction techniques, verbal and nonverbal effects, and the relative influence of the methodologies of the various psychotherapeutic schools. Any evaluation of the results of psychotherapy naturally has to give great weight to the assessment of these and other intrinsic factors. As difficult as the consideration of these elements is, the weighting of *extrinsic* factors for their influence upon the psychotherapeutic process is even more complex. The extrinsic factors are variables which operate upon the process outside of the one-to-one setting. These constitute a variety of influences which have a bearing upon either the patient or the therapist or both outside of the therapeutic session. Their relevance is difficult and complex because as influential variables they are elusive, multidimensional, and even more difficult to control than the intrinsic ones.

A comparison of these two sets of factors presents us on the one hand, for example, relative to the intrinsic ones, with the conditions of a series of therapeutic sessions. Each of these can be viewed as a time sample in a relatively consistent setting narrowed down to the interaction between two persons. They can be assessed for content, interaction, process, movement, sequential order, or other parameters in which the raw data are subject to collection by written, visual, auditory, or electronic means. As complex as this procedure is it is at least narrowed and controlled to an extent. On the other hand, the identification and collection of raw data associated with the extrinsic variables must take into account the broad spectrum of a 24-hour day in a variety of settings with a multitude of individuals in contact with the patient and with the doctor singly or in groups. The methodologic considerations involved in evaluating these influences where control is so difficult are inordinately complex.

This presentation is concerned primarily with a consideration of the extrinsic factors in the evaluation of the results of psychotherapy because these variables lend themselves to some degree of control in the inpatient setting. Here a small number of patients can be observed over a length of time by a staff focused upon suitable and particularized observations at all levels throughout the 24-hour day. Since any evaluation of the results of psychotherapy must deal concurrently with the assessment of both intrinsic and extrinsic variables, studies on the intrinsic ones are currently being carried out at the hospital under a grant from the National Institute of Mental Health and will be the subject of later papers. This paper concerns itself with preliminary considerations of the extrinsic factors which seem to us to have a bearing upon the process of psychotherapy in the inpatient setting.

We begin with a theoretical framework which allows us to identify upon what levels we are evaluating. An activity may be evaluated on a basis of one or more levels or types of measurements based on different value systems:[1]

> At the first level, evaluation is an estimate which an individual or group places on an activity or service—what it means to the recipients according to their own value system.
>
> At the second level, evaluation is the appraised worth; that is, a value placed on an activity or service after a reasonable examination and after the appraisers have compared it with other services. It is presumed that these appraisers have had experience in their respective fields; the criteria are empiric and based on subjective judgment.
>
> The third level is that of scientific measurement—an expression of value when measured against accepted standardized procedures. . . . In general terms, any study evaluated by the rigorous methods of scientific measurement should adhere to such principles as formulation of the problem, careful planning of research design, delineation of methods of data collection, and logical analysis of experimental results.

In the evaluation of psychotherapeutic results in terms of the extrinsic variables at work, this particular project has functioned on the second and third levels of the evaluation method. It has been carried out predominantly by a group of investigators who by consensual validation have worked toward hypotheses from conclusions drawn from their observations as experts. But at the same time a beginning was made in scientific measurement by statistically collating data about the patient census and treatment process.

Methodologic considerations in assessing any mental health activity should pursue one or more of the following steps in evaluation as set forth by French:[2] 1. Identification of the goals to be sought or measured; 2. analysis of the problems with which the activity must cope; 3. description and standardization of the activity; 4. measurement of the degree of change that takes place; 5. determination as to whether the change observed is the result of the activity or due to some other cause; and 6. some indication of the durability of the effects.

This preliminary study of ours concerns itself particularly with step 5, wherein hypotheses relating to extrinsic variables are formulated in terms of whether changes observed supposed to be the result of psychotherapy are "the result of that activity or due to some other cause."

In order to proceed with step 5 (to determine whether changes are the result of psychotherapy or due to some other cause) additional methodologic factors have to be considered. These include 1. control of variables, 2. selective perception, 3. the cumulative effects, 4. concurrent countereffects, 5. concurrent parallel effects, and 6. the prospective utilization of control groups.[3] We will now elaborate on these methodologic factors.

CONTROL OF VARIABLES

In any situation involving human behavior, numerous variables are of influence. Where interaction between individuals and groups are concerned, variables impinge upon the situation with different weights. All possible factors which have any relevance to the outcome of a situation should be identified and weighted for their effect in any evaluation effort. This is necessary not only to true assessment, but serves methodologically as a safeguard against erroneous conclusions and interpretations drawn as to cause and effect. Standen's ludicrous example illustrates this point[4]

There will be an argument that, in principle, runs like this: A man gets drunk on Monday on whisky and soda water; he gets drunk on Tuesday on brandy and soda water, and on Wednesday on gin and soda water. What caused his drunkenness? Obviously, the common factor, the soda water.

The identification and weighting of variables means *control of variables* to insure validity in evaluation.[5] This is essential in the assessment of the results of psychotherapy where claims can be so easily made upon opinion and values. To sharpen controls we classify influential factors as *patent variables* and *hidden variables*. By patent variables we identify those factors which are general and universal and which might obviously be assigned in any demographic study. These would include in our context age of patient, sex of patient, geographic origin of patient population, socioeconomic status, duration of illness, previous hospitalizations, previous treatment diagnosis, and administration of drugs. Such patent variables lend themselves more easily than the hidden ones to statistical analysis. For this reason we began to explore statistical assessment in this study of 500 cases.

The hidden variables are the elusive ones. As external variables acting upon the psychotherapeutic process they are largely relationship factors operating between the patient and the therapist and the patient and other individuals and groups outside of the treatment hour. They are, therefore, difficult to measure and must be assessed by a variety of methods often differing from the statistical one. They must first be identified as possibilities by consensual validation, treated as hypotheses and then tested. Examples of such hidden variables are selection of the patient population, personality characteristics of department heads, influence of removal of patient from stressful situations at home, effect of the therapeutic community, influence of patients upon the patient assessed, effects of family therapy, staff conferences, and visiting policies, communication practices of psychiatric aides, impact of the nationality of therapist, and other factors.

SELECTIVE PERCEPTION

In the evaluation of psychotherapy or of any other form of mental health activity, particular attention must be given to the selective perception of the evaluators. The tendency to categorize data according to prevalent theories of human behavior or from the administrative goals and policies of an institution must be taken into account. Such hidden factors as the importance assigned to psychotherapy, emphasis upon dynamic formulation, selective interest in the Freudian theoretical model, concern for the concept of the therapeutic community, necessity of public relations, and priority of interests (psychotherapy, countertransference, electro-shock therapy) are among the external variables which must be protected from the errors inherent in selective perception. Such errors are guarded against by consensual validation in the institutional setting.

CUMULATIVE EFFECTS

Variables may cluster and have an accumulative effect which individually may not have as much influence. For instance, the combination of factors such as a staff of psychiatric aides functioning on a closed ward with the factor of patients who have little cohesiveness as a group and who, as an additional factor, have fewer visitors than other patients—all of these together may have a cumulative influence on the results of psychotherapy which is more telling than such factors as the age of the patients or of the aides.

CONCURRENT COUNTEREFFECTS

Certain stimuli or situations may spontaneously serve to counteract the goals or effects of psychotherapy or may lend themselves for selection by the patient in his efforts to resist psychotherapy. These can be so prevalent that continuous screening for them has to be performed by evaluators. Cases in point would include an awareness of the negating effects of visits away from the hospital in certain instances versus the results of psychotherapy at any given time, and the possibility that a traditional nursing activity might happen to oppose a planned psychotherapeutic goal. Even a group activity or its absence may induce a concurrent countereffect.

CONCURRENT PARALLEL EFFECTS

Variables may act synergistically to produce an effect which is greater than their sum or individual value. For instance, with certain patients the situations already delineated as examples of countereffects may serve to give concurrent parallel results. The results of psychotherapy rated as excellent may have reached this level because the patient was visiting at home on weekends, whereas therapy would have been less effective without visits. The validity of the psychotherapy itself must then be weighed in the light of the parallel effects of the extraneous hidden factor of home visiting. The possible parallel effects of drugs or even of housekeeping practices within the hospital must be taken into consideration.

CONTROL GROUPS

A thoughtful research design requires that measured changes in a group under study be compared with a control group not exposed to the activity being measured. In any long-range plan to evaluate the results of psychotherapy this must be given the utmost consideration. Because *all* patients at High Point Hospital are exposed to three psychotherapy hours per week, this factor remains in the broadest sense a constant one. Being constant this has a value against which can be measured the effects of diverse intrinsic and extrinsic variables. Moreover, there are built-in control groups in the form of standardized patient groupings, according to extent of convalescence, which can be compared for the effects of variables on them.

The establishment of traditional control groups in which no psychotherapy at all would be administered has been considered by us. This attempt has been delayed because of the difficulties inherent in a clinical program in which optimal care of the patient takes precedence over all other activities. It is our expectation that such a plan of control will be initiated at a future stage of study. Consideration is also being given to an action research endeavor in which patent variables could be manipulated, namely, treating one group of patients under psychotherapy concurrently with drugs, while a second group would receive no chemotherapeutic agents whatsoever.

SOME SIGNIFICANT EXTRINSIC VARIABLES

In addition to the significance of psychotherapy, experience in our particular hospital indicates the likely importance of many variables to the ultimate result achieved with a patient. This becomes increasingly evident as data are collected and studied. A number of these variables, both patent and hidden, have already been mentioned and several, which would seem to require special consideration in our own attempt to evaluate the results of psychotherapy, will be elaborated. It is our hope that we may ultimately subject these variables, which we hypothesize to be significant, to a planned study.

The selection of a type of patient for any inpatient program will contribute to the end results achieved. This would seem particularly true where analytically-oriented psychotherapy is emphasized. In addition to the patent variables involved—such as age, sex, duration of illness, diagnosis—there are hidden variables such as motivation, the nature and effect of previous psychotherapeutic treatment, the patient's leading personality drives, and the patient's perception of the hospital environment. Many others may be surmised. All of them will have some effect on outcome, and the weight of the psychotherapeutic process itself is thereby more difficult to determine. Once these variables are identified and their significance to the ultimate outcome known, selection of patients for analytic psychotherapy may in turn be more precise and the results of psychotherapy thereby improved. Meanwhile we must remain somewhat critical in evaluating the results of psychotherapy.

Each hospital will have its own known, as well as obscure, criteria for the selection of patients. Although much will depend on the nature of its treatment program, other determining factors will also be present. The smaller the bed capacity, and the more defined the therapeutic program, the more exact and defined would be the factors deciding patient selection. In our own particular case, the census is limited to 45 patients housed on two floors of one modest-sized building. The patients accordingly live together in close proximity for rather extended periods of time. The ability of a patient to "fit in" with the general group must, therefore, be taken into account. Since analytically-oriented psychotherapy, supported by drug therapy, family therapy and a therapeutic community structure, is *the* mode of therapy, patients will be selected mainly with these facts in mind. Accordingly, organic and relatively old patients will be excluded. Patients whose histories suggest a better prognosis when exposed to our therapeutic armamentarium will tend to be selected. Here factors such as the psychiatrist's need to gain the personal satisfaction and professional prestige forthcoming from "good results" may also help determine patient selection.

Patients with a more guarded prognosis will not be

excluded although they will be limited in number. The effect of such patients upon each other as they may affect results will be weighed in selecting them for admission. The duration of illness, nature of symptoms, and level of intelligence will be considered as they may affect prognosis and length of hospitalization. Since short hospitalization is now in vogue, and the quality of the therapist's performance is judged by the length of time patients remain in the hospital, the tendency is to select those who will respond rapidly.* Where costs are a factor, this point will contribute to the selection of the patient and of the hospital by the patient. Unfortunately, the economic factor is too significant today in the voluntary and public as well as proprietary hospital.

Although age, per se, is a patent extrinsic variable, the proportion of adolescents in the hospital at any one time in relation to the adults will determine much of what is afoot among the patients because of the well-known catalytic effect of adolescents. Accordingly, this factor is now a hidden extrinsic variable which will affect results because we select a fair number of adolescents.

At High Point Hospital, we maintain a relatively optimistic therapeutic attitude toward schizophrenic patients. Accordingly, we select them freely, and do not shrink from making the diagnosis of schizophrenia when it is at all apparent. Their presence in large numbers, of course, will affect psychotherapeutic results. Again, although diagnosis, per se, is a patent variable, the proportion and type of schizophrenics present in the patient population at any one time

* Presently in psychiatry there is an unfortunate tendency to equate "good results" with length of hospitalization. This is true in every type of institution from public to voluntary to proprietary. As a matter of fact, sometimes it would seem as though there were an unholy competition to see which hospital is maintaining a shorter average length of hospital stay. Our less than objective criteria for discharging a patient, let alone assessing his status at the time of release, do not, of course, ease our problem. It would seem that much more reliable and adequate criteria have yet to be found for evaluating the results of any therapy, particularly those of psychotherapy, than length of hospitalization and elapsed time before readmission.

will affect general atmosphere, and accordingly be acting as a hidden variable.

The Psychotherapeutic Community: The hospital environment in which a patient is immersed may be as important a factor in his recuperation as is the fact that he has been removed from his stressful home surroundings. Accordingly, at High Point, we try to construct and maintain a social structure that is an integral part of the therapeutic program. We recognize that the term "therapeutic community" is used all too loosely and that the characteristics of this "community" are hardly ever defined objectively. Further, at High Point Hospital we have begun to talk of ourselves as a "psychotherapeutic community" if only to present ourselves with the necessity of defining and justifying the proper use of the term.

In essence, we maintain a tightly integrated social structure in which patients and personnel are not only bound by good hospital practices, but by the hospital's laws, values, and mores. The medical staff works as a team and is the chief authority. It is assisted professionally by the nursing and social group work departments, which broaden out the treatment team. The patient's role is defined by his involvement in the fabric of the hospital through participation in committees which have work and responsibilities socially useful to the hospital population. The extent and nature of the patient's participation is prescribed by the medical team. This is done in keeping with his present problems and potential for growth through interactivity with other patients and with personnel on the broader treatment team. Because of a highly coordinated communication system, no aspect of the patient's hospital life is unknown to the medical team. This includes his behavior and participation in the one-to-one psychotherapeutic relationship, which is also exposed to the weekly team conferences.

Time does not permit me to say more about this complex set of hidden variables subsumed under the term psychotherapeutic community, except that we are convinced it is a factor which must be more scientifically studied and weighed in the balance when evaluating psychotherapeutic results, at least at High Point Hospital. It provides a third dimension of significance to the psychotherapeutic result by exposing the patient to numerous relationship factors other that the formal doctor-patient one.

Family Therapy: At our hospital, significant family members are involved in conjoint therapeutic sessions once weekly for indefinite periods at some strategic time during the patient's stay. Time does not permit us to go into greater detail except to say that family involvement has both negative and positive effects on the patient's course. Over all it improves communication between family, patient, and therapist. Again, in a dynamic manner, it expands the relationship factors to which the patient is exposed. These are of such an intricate and moving nature that we feel they cannot help but be affecting the psychotherapeutic result. Accordingly, family therapy as we use it becomes another hidden variable which must be exposed to a planned study and ultimately weighed in the scale.

CONCLUSIONS

A psychiatric inpatient program based on a foundation of intensive analytically oriented psychotherapy has developed into a highly complex social structure with many facets which influence the course of patients. It has seemed necessary, therefore, to establish an ongoing evaluation of the results of this fundamental policy of intensive psychotherapy for every patient. In the total program which has evolved, we have had to scrutinize our basic assumption that the single most important ingredient in the care of hospitalized psychiatric patients is structured individual psychotherapy.

Such evaluation, however, is admittedly difficult, for all of the aspects of the program must be acknowledged if the validity of any one of them is to be ultimately assured. In our study of 500 cases we first endeavored to look at some of the factors which must be considered. Our attempt led us to discuss some of the components of methodology which must be honored in any evaluation study of psychotherapy, particularly in the inpatient setting.

Our deliberations led primarily to the consideration of several variables which must be identified and weighted. We have distinguished *intrinsic variables* which operate in the one-to-one setting from the *extrinsic ones* which refer to relationships for both the patient and the therapist outside the psychotherapeutic session. In this paper, our principle concern has been with those extrinsic factors which are constantly at play within the therapeutic milieu. We have made a preliminary and tentative effort to study statistically the traditional patent variables. In the process, however, we were impressed by the need to consider certain categories of variables which could clarify the evaluation effort, rather than by the urge to emphasize statistics.

We conclude that within the extrinsic variables are hidden or elusive ones which utimately require the most refined screening to safeguard the sound evaluation of psychotherapy. We have pointed out the character of some of the principal hidden variables which must be identified and weighted in any hospital setting where psychotherapy is systematically conducted. We have focused upon three particularly: the selection of patients, the psychotherapeutic community structure, and the conduct of family therapy. At High Point Hosital these have had particular relevance to our considerations. In other hospitals, perhaps, different variables will have higher priority. It may be that universal categories of variables must be considered in any attempt to assess the results of psychotherapy. Further studies from this and other inpatient settings are indicated to assure the validity of this hypothesis.

REFERENCES

1. Southard, C. G.: *Symposium on the Evaluation of Community Mental Health Programs.* National Institute of Mental Health, 1952-1953 Seminar Series, November 25, 1952. Unpublished Discussions.

2. French, D. G.: *An Approach to Measuring Results in Social Work.* Columbia University Press, New York, 1952.
3. *Evaluation in Mental Health.* Report of the Subcommittee on Evaluation of Mental Health Activities. U. S. Department of Health, Education and Welfare. Public Health Service Publication No. 413. U. S. Government Printing Office, Washington, D. C.
4. Standen, A.: *Science Is a Sacred Cow.* E. P. Dutton, New York, 1950
5. Burnett, F. M. and Greenhill, M. H.: Some Problems in the Evaluation of an Inservice Training Program in Mental Health. *Am. J. Publ. Health,* 44: 12, 1954.

5

Changing Relation of the Patient, Family and Practicing Psychiatrist to the Therapeutic Community

ALEXANDER GRALNICK, M.D.

HAVING COME THROUGH several decades of rather productive changes, we are currently living in the midst of exciting times within our specialty. The introduction of insulin therapy[1] infused us with an optimism from which we have never quite receded. It is true that innovations have arrived with such frequency since then that there has not been time to return to any degree of lethargy or pessimism. Electroshock therapy[2] aroused any flagging enthusiasm which may have stolen upon us when insulin therapy did not continue to meet up to our anticipations, as did its various modifications, and combinations of it with insulin coma treatment. Metrazol convulsive therapy had already come and gone, and carbon dioxide inhalation therapy and intravenous ether drip therapy also saw their day, and night. Where the effects of the physiological procedure itself did not seem sufficient to explain the improvement in patients, additional psychotherapeutic aspects of them were described.[3-8]

Cerebral surgery entered the picture to handle those patients who did not respond to our numerous ministrations, but instead remained the dregs of a rather bitter cup. Psychosurgery became our answer to the remnant of psychotics

Reprinted from Denber, H. C. B. et al., *Research Conference on Therapeutic Community,* pp. 153-162, 1959, Charles C Thomas, Publisher, Springfield, Illinois.

who resisted our march forward, and frustrated our ego satisfaction. Then, as though there could be sensed some seed of misgiving with the results of these procedures, the drug therapies came upon the scene. And now, psychopharmacology[9] is all the rage, and miracle drugs, tranquilizers and psychic energizers command our attention as we coin new words to explain our new comprehension, cover our yet remaining ignorance, or mask our chagrin.

As though all of this were not enough, we have also had our share of innovations on the non-physiological side. Witness the changing attitudes in psychoanalysis[10] and the increasing influence of allied disciplines in psychiatry. The growth of group therapy and family therapy[11] are also illustrative, as is the growing field of psychosomatic medicine. The increasing tendency to ambulate patients as rapidly as possible is in part a response to economic pressures, but also an evidence of belief in its preferability to inpatient care. In other words, the patient is thought to be benefited if he is out of the hospital as soon as possible. The growth of psychiatric units within general hospitals is an obvious response to economic factors, and to the belief that patients should be brought closer to medicine, to the family and community. Such innovations as the day-hospital, night-hospital and the open door policy are similar evidences of our efforts to improve treatment of the mentally ill. Although the above list is by no means complete, we may add "and not lastly the concept of the therapeutic community" which, although not an entirely new idea, seems to be coming increasingly to the fore.[12-15]

At various stages of his knowledge man deals with problems differently. He has not always treated the mentally ill by institutionalization as he has in the last century or so. At first we hospitalized the patient to merely remove him from society and prevent him from doing injury. It is true that the early primitive methods were supplanted by more humane attitudes and procedures, perhaps to compensate the poor inmate for that of which he had been deprived, and possibly to assuage our own guilt feelings for denying him society's pleasures. This did not indicate that we believed the kindlier treatment necessarily had therapeutic value.

In more recent years we have devoted our major attention to active treatment, research and theory. Essentially this has meant an acting upon the patient through some type of physiological procedure designed to restore his equilibrium. In some instances, intervention has been principally through psychotherapy, with the physiological actually subordinated to it.

As horizons have been expanded we have come to look upon the hospital not as "good" or "bad" in which the "right" or "wrong" treatment is given, but as a community with its own social structure. As such, it immediately suggests overtones of a therapeutic nature. In such a setting all of the participants take on a human quality, that of interacting beings who affect each other in a vital way. Much more is involved than the mere giving of a drug or application of a procedure, and the doctor is more than a technician. He too is not exempt from scrutiny, and his personal qualities and emotions become as significant as his knowledge and ability.

The relation of the patient, family and referring psychiatrist to the hospital has been rather well known. Essentially the patient has been the unwilling participant, committed by legal means, ejected from his social setting to become a cog in the machinery of the large institution, and acted upon by doctors in an effort to repair him so that he may be restored to society. If occupied during his stay it is with the object of keeping him busy and out of mischief. Therapeutic aspects of such occupation are in terms of ego satisfaction in manual accomplishments and competitive sports, or in terms of improvement automatic to mental diversion.

By and large, the patient's family has had little significant relationship to the institution. Essentially the relative has been a source of historical information, a visitor, and perhaps the haven to whom the doctor will return the patient. This has been true for two likely reasons. First, that staff shortages have made it impossible to devote much time to the relative, and second, that our basic theory has branded him the villain of the piece. Consequently, he is separated off from the patient and a certain degree of ill-will is borne him by the psychiatrist in the protective role he assumes vis-a-vis the patient. For both reasons, of course, the psychiatrist's experience in developing an active role for the relative has been limited, and his ability to integrate him into the therapeutic program has been kept at a minimum. Freud has expressed our general despair in this area by stating, "As for treatment of the relative I must confess myself utterly at a loss, and I have altogether little faith in any individual treatment of them."[16] However, more recently, a more optimistic and realistic approach to the family is being taken as we develop our thinking about the therapeutic community.[17-19]

The bulk of psychiatrists in the community have had the barest relationship to the mental institution, other than to recommend hospitalization when they can no longer manage patients otherwise. In most cases such recommendation is made under emergency rather than elective conditions. The usual conscientious doctor dislikes giving up, and perhaps admitting defeat. In psychiatry particularly we look upon separating the patient from his physician as especially traumatic, and therefore inadvisable. This too would encourage the therapist to cling to the bitter end. Naturally, the crowded conditions, poor staffing, and limited therapeutic program of our institutions have not given the practicing psychiatrist much encouragement to advise hospitalization too readily. His attitude toward the hospital psychiatrist is perhaps a factor too. Of course, the public's attitude toward hospitalization and the patient's resistance to it constantly limit the psychiatrist from advising it any too soon. It is a fact too that the criteria for recommending hospitalization are not any too clear. Most unfortunate is the fact that once hospitalized, contact between patient and therapist is generally completely severed, although in some cases this may be a good thing. Basically then, a vacuum exists between the private psychiatrist and the mental institution.

When we think of the hospital as a therapeutic community we tend to emphasize the significance of its social structure as a therapeutic force. This concept suggests that treatment procedures and drugs do not alone make the advanced hospital, but that the nature of the social relationships existing therein are perhaps quite as important.[20-22] If we are to understand the significance of the therapeutic community we must first attempt its adequate description.

It is taken for granted firstly that the therapeutic community will adequately tend to the physical and physiological requirements of its patients. Over and above this, however, the basic approach of its medical staff toward mental disease will be most important. The physician will treat the patient as a person who has a disease. He will not be treating a disease within a patient. With this approach the needs of the individual as such, and the group of which he is a part, will receive equitable management, as their interests tend to clash. The team-approach would also seem to be an integral part of a therapeutic community, as would the opportunity for close relationship between the patient and his therapist. The doctor should have the opportunity to deal with both the therapeutic and administrative aspects of his patient's management. The medical staff, dynamically oriented, should make hospital and therapeutic policy. Patients should have an opportunity to work closely together in activities designed to contribute to the social setting in which they are living. The units of a therapeutic community will have to be small if an atmosphere of intimacy is to develop. Policy should be flexible and designed to meet changing conditions, and means of communication among patients, and between patients and staff, should be of the best.[23] Value judgments must find a place in the therapeutic community if structure and order in its social relationships are to be maintained.

THE THERAPEUTIC COMMUNITY

It is a social structure with its own particular ways and laws, and is not to be confused with a setting in which one has freedom to do as he pleases without restriction. It has conscious design, and its main aim is to help the patient to become a more mature and rational person, not merely as well as he once was. It is not necessarily designed for speed of recovery and to meet the requirements of limited budgets.

Although the concept and the full description of the therapeutic community have yet to be detailed, we know enough to realize that all concerned are faced with changing relationships to the mental institution. The hospital psychiatrist has been facing this wherever his organization has been moving in the new direction. But what of the others?

When the prospective patient realizes that in the newer atmosphere he is a respected individual of the hospital community, not "the patient" and that he has a significant role in its fabric, he will be more apt to accept hospitalization. It may be expected too that he will welcome staying in the more wholesome atmosphere which offers him more promise, and gain the most from what it has to offer him. We may anticipate further that the changed conditions will help dissipate the feelings of shame and of social stigma which surround hospitalization today. Above all, the patient should have a much healthier respect for the hospital and fellow patients, and be a contributing participant to its welfare, even perhaps after he has left its confines.[24]

It is likely that the true therapeutic community will enlist the relative more actively in its program.[25] Signs of this are already evident in the group meetings being held with relatives. Authority figures within the hospital will establish parental relationships to patients. Under such conditions they will develop more sympathetic understanding of the problems of the true parents and relatives. Working relationships between therapist and relatives on behalf of the patient should then improve. More wholesome attitudes on the part of relatives toward our institutions should encourage them to influence governmental agencies in favor of better treatment and research programs. In the therapeutic community the therapist will give the relative more understanding of psychopathology so that he may more thoroughly comprehend the patient. Relatives will appreciate this and in turn will be seen as less villainous.

As mental institutions have become more active treatment centers the practicing psychiatrist has increasingly viewed them with favor. Any reservations have been a reflection of the manner in which patients as people are treated because of overcrowded conditions. Among other things, the rapid growth of small psychiatric units within general hospitals is a sign of such dissatisfaction. In such units the practicing psychiatrist maintains closer and continuing contact with his patient in a more wholesome setting. It is to be expected, however, that as our institutions develop into therapeutic communities the psychiatrist will alter his attitudes, and thereby help affect the negative attitudes of the public. It is to be hoped that he may take a more active role in both the training and treatment programs of our larger institutions, and thereby promote their growth into better therapeutic communities. The practicing psychiatrists' participation in the treatment of hospitalized patients may ultimately be considered an ingredient of the therapeutic community concept. There was a time when state institutions were quite isolated geographically. What must be overcome now is the emotional isolation in which they have been maintained. At any rate, the practicing psychiatrist is faced with an increasing challenge as the therapeutic community develops within institutions.

We are living in a time when great pressures, emotional and economic, are being exerted to have us produce quick results in psychiatry. Progress is being measured by the rapidity with which we can get patients out of our hospitals, as if being out is the sine qua non of being well. It would be as though some magic is worked once a patient walks out of the front door of an institution, or some worthy service is done the patient if he is saved from entering a hospital, no matter how long he may otherwise be kept in a state of imbalance or unresolved conflict. Improved mental health in a community seems to be measured by a decreasing state budget and the brevity of the average hospital stay.

Under such conditions perspective and the true interest of science may be easily lost. We do not tend to engage in this type of thinking in physical medicine. What if we did with cancer? It is not necessarily serving the best interests of society or of patients themselves to have an increasing number of mentally sick people walking about. Time, of course, will help us with any such evaluation. We may find yet that the answer will remain in relatively long hospitalization, but under the better conditions of a therapeutic community.

Of course, logic would seem to suggest that if mental illness is even in part socially determined,[26-29] then favorable results would flow from the more rational social structure of the therapeutic community. Knitting the hospital as such more closely into the larger community would also seem to foretell more favorable results. In many ways, however, the therapeutic community calls for a more complicated social organization for the hospital, with more integrated and complex activity programs of patient participation in the institution's fabric. It may suggest and require longer hospitalizations for the reconstruction of patients. Many may oppose any such trend. It has already been said that activity and occupational programs should be cut down out of fear that they promote comfort and prolong stays. We should beware of pressures which, in the service of economy, would curtail the logical and scientific growth of the therapeutic community concept. At the same time, caution is needed in evaluating this newer concept of treatment. The "new" is not necessarily the "best" or even the "better." Wholesome development and rational change in our system of hospital treatment would seem necessary, but let us beware of discarding the baby with the bathwater.

SUMMARY AND CONCLUSION

The changing scene in psychiatric hospitals has been described with emphasis on the relationship between psychiatrist, patient and family. It is believed that emphasis must be shifted towards "total" treatment of the patient in an enlightened social setting. Here, active patient participation will be an index of healthy group interaction between various staff members and patients.

The private psychiatrist should be integrated into the hospital activities.

The therapeutic effectiveness of short versus long hospitalization has been considered.

BIBLIOGRAHY

1. Gralnick, A.: A seven year survey of insulin treatment in schizophrenia. *Am. J. Psychiat., 101:* 449, 1945.
2. Gralnick, A.: A three year survey of electroshock therapy: Report on 276 cases; comparative value of insulin coma therapy. *Am. J. Psychiat., 102:* 583, 1946.
3. Gralnick, A.: Psychotherapeutic and interpersonal aspects of insulin treatment. *Psychiat. Quart., 18:* 179, 1944.
4. Kalinowsky, L. B.: Problems of psychotherapy and transference in shock treatments and psychosurgery. *Psychosom. Med., 18:* 399, 1956.
5. Hill, L. B., and Patton, J. D.: When physical therapy (shock) facilitates psychotherapy. *Am. J. Psychiat., 113:* 60, 1956.
6. Silverberg, W. V., and Hirning, L. D.: Psychotherapy and adjunctive means in psychiatry. *Am. J. Psychother., 12:* 760, 1958.
7. Rabiner, E. L., and Gralnick, A.: Transference and countertransference phenomena in choice of shock: A review of 108 cases with a comparative study. *A.M.A. Arch. Neurol. Psychiat. 81,* April 1959.
8. Gralnick, A.: *Adjunctive Shock Treatment in an Intensive Psychotherapeutic Program.* 2nd International Congress of Psychiatry, Vol. 2, p. 380, Zurich, Orell, Füssli Arts Graphiques, 1959.
9. Kline, N. S., Ed.: *Psychopharmacology Frontiers.* Boston, Little, Brown & Co., 1959.
10. Mohr, G. J.: *Psychoanalysis: Some Present Day Assessments.* Academy of Psychoanalysis, New York, 1958.
11. Ackerman, N. W.: Toward an integrative therapy of the family. *Am. J. Psychiat., 114:* 727, 1958.

12. MacDonald, J. M., and Daniels, M. L.: The psychiatric ward as a therapeutic community. *J. Nerv. Ment. Dis., 124:* 148, 1956.
13. Jones, M.: The treatment of personality disorders in a therapeutic community. *Psychiatry, 20:* 211, 1957.
14. Wilmer, H. A.: Toward a definition of the therapeutic community. *Am. J. Psychiat., 114:* 824, 1958.
15. Gralnick, A.: Behavioral determinants in a therapeutic milieu. In: *The Dynamics of Psychiatric Drug Therapy.* Ed. Sarwer-Foner, G. J., Springfield, Charles C Thomas, 1959.
16. Freud, S.: Recommendations for physicians on the psychoanalytic method of treatment. *Collected Papers, 2:* 323, London, Hogarth Press, 1933.
17. Hall, B. H., and Wheeler, W.: The patient and his relatives. *Social Work, 2:* 75, 1957.
18. Lefebvre, P., Atkins, J., Duckman, J. and Gralnick, A.: The role of the relative in a psychotherapeutic program. *J. Canad. Psychiat. Assoc., 3:* 110, 1958.
19. Gralnick, A.: The family in psychotherapy. In: *Individual and Family Dynamics.* Ed. Masserman, J., New York, Grune & Stratton, 1959
20. Gralnick, A., Schacht, M., and Kempster, S. W.: Psychotherapy in a private mental hospital. *Am. J. Psychoth., 8:* 312, 1954.
21. Starr, A., Gralnick, A.: Factors determining the initial effect of hospitalization on cases of schizophrenia. *Am. J. Psychoth., 9:* 243, 1955.
22. Cohen, R. A.: The hospital as a therapeutic instrument. *Psychiatry, 21:* 29, 1958.
23. O'Connor, W., Carstairs, G. M., and Rawnsley, K.: Communication in a mental hospital population. *Int. J. Soc. Psychiat., 3:* 183, 1957.
24. Gralnick, A., and D'Elia, F.: *Role of the Patient in the Therapeutic Community: Patient-participation.* Southern Divisional Meeting, American Psychiatric Assoc., Miami, 1958.
25. Gralnick, A.: Relation of the family to a psychotherapeutic inpatient program. *Int. J. Soc. Psychiat.* V: 2, 1959.
26. Gralnick, A.: Folie à deux—The psychosis of association. *Psychiat. Quart., 16:* 230 and 491, 1942.
27. Gralnick, A.: The Carrington family: A psychiatric and social study illustrating the psychosis of association or folie à deux. *Psychiat. Quart., 17:* 294, 1943.
28. Gruenberg, E. M.: Socially shared psychopathology. In: *Explorations in Social Psychiatry,* New York, Basic Books, 1958.
29. Redlich, F. D.: Social aspects of psychotherapy in the United States. *Progress in Psychotherapy,* 3:79, 1958, New York, Grune & Stratton.

DISCUSSION OF DR. GRALNICK'S PAPER

Dr. Max Fink:

I would agree that there is no one "therapeutic community" but that all hospital aggregates are "communities" and the therapeutic element is a matter of degree. This conference has as a title a single concept, "Therapeutic Community" and I would like to change it to "Therapeutic Communities." The discussion today, I believe, has suffered from a lack of discrimination of the individual differences in population. It seems as if the recommendations for one population should be applicable to another. But this is not true. The experiments of Drs. Sullivan and Freida Fromm-Reichman were limited to severe schizophrenic patients. Other discussants have described groups which are differently constituted, such as the emphasis on psychopathic personalities in the Jones' community or the chronic group of patients seen at Boston Psychopathic. I would like to make a plea that the discussion be focused on some of the differences in population and the extent to which such differences affect the ability with which such changes in milieu augment or depress therapeusis.

6

On Behavioral Determinants in a Therapeutic Milieu

ALEXANDER GRALNICK, M.D.

THROUGH THE YEARS, and into the current era, psychiatrists within and without mental institutions have varied greatly in their approach to the management and treatment of the mentally ill. We are all too well aware of this fact for it to be more than mentioned. It is largely true, too, that the greater portion of psychiatrists' energies have been devoted to an exploration of the biochemical origins and physiological treatment of mental illness. This conference is an encouraging occasion, particularly as it flies in the face of pressure to push the more popular approach. The title of this conference would, at the least, suggest that psychological and sociological factors are of significance—if not of major importance—in the administration of an effective medication. It is especially gratifying that such an international symposium is convened so early in our experience with the neuroleptic, or tranquilizing drugs. I believe that this is a good sign and indicates that psychiatrists have learned something in the last generation. I do not remember that any similar meeting was held after the introduction of insulin and electro-shock therapy. As a matter of fact, I may be correct in stating that no such conference relative to these physical therapies has ever been held. I do recall that those of us who

Reprinted from *The Dynamics of Psychiatric Drug Therapy*, edited by G. J. Sarwer-Foner, M.D., pp. 153-162, Charles C Thomas, 1959.

did speak out early about the psychological and sociological aspects of shock treatment were few, were paid relatively little heed, and were but small voices among a rising crescendo of expressions of optimism at the startling results achieved by shock treatment. It was as though our problem had been solved.

This particular conference is a reflection of more sober thinking in psychiatry. Additional ones may further brake any unhealthy trend of unwarranted optimism, and promote a more balanced approach in theorization, treatment and research. Much credit is due those who have had the fortitude to convene us, and labored to afford us this opportunity.

It is generally believed that in addition to constitutional factors the milieu in which one is conceived and into which he is born largely determines the nature of the personality and behavior. The environment in which one is reared exerts innumerable influences which mold the emotions and establish the attitudes with which one, in turn, deals with the experiences of life. Under certain conditions of stress a human being may develop so differently from his fellow men that he can no longer live with them under usual circumstances. He develops a pattern of mental, emotional and behavioral life which we term psychotic. Ultimately, this unfortunate person may be lodged in a mental institution which will attempt to repair the damage done him.

Through the ages man dealt with this problem in a variety of ways. He has managed the mentally ill variously, but in the more recent history of their treatment mainly by the process of institutionalization. This may not be true forever. The former half of this period of history was devoted chiefly to custodial care, whereas the more current part has been devoted more exclusively to scientific research, theorization, and treatment. In both portions of this era the general thinking has been that the patient be removed from society. In the former portion that he be removed to prevent him from injuring society, and in the latter portion that the patient be confined for general care and treatment.

While this is not an exact presentation of things, and custodial care is still more prevalent than we would like it to be, the description is sufficiently accurate as a basis for this discussion.

Essentially, treatment has meant, in addition to humane management, a kind of acting upon the patient through medication or one form of physiological procedure or another, designed to affect his economy and restore his balance. While this has been the prevailing approach, in some few instances treatment has meant intervention principally through the process of psychotherapy (occasionally psychoanalytically oriented, but more generally not), with physiological procedures really subordinated to it. In decidedly more instances, where psychotherapy is used it is the *handmaid* of the physiological approach. In relatively few institutions is it the abiding faith of its medical staff that psychotherapy is as significant as, if not more so than, any other therapeutic procedure.

It is the burgeoning of the psychotherapeutic approach that gives rise to the prevailing terminology that appears on the orientation sheet that was sent us about this conference. The word physiological appears only twice, whereas milieu, sociological determinants, personality, motivations, transference and countertransference are prevalent—the terms associated with an appreciation of the significance of human interaction in any treatment procedure in psychiatry.

In more recent years consideration has been given to the idea that the hospital is a community. As such it should be subject to searching exploration to determine its social structure and effects on the patient. It has been suggested that as a community it be constructed to be as therapeutic as possible—that it be a therapeutic community. This concept is quite different from the one to which we are accustomed, namely, that we have a "good" hospital in which the proper medication is given in the correct dosages or the appropriate shock treatment is given in sufficient numbers.

This newer concept indicates that neither physiological nor psychotherapeutic procedures of and by themselves are important, but that the social relationships within the hospital are. It opens an entirely new vista, raises a host of new questions, and opens entirely new areas of investigation. It indicates that the patient need not be thought of as being removed from society, but as being removed to a society subject to study and regulation under conditions reasonably controlled by psychiatrists. It may expose the patient to exactly the same pressure and interactions as elsewhere, but more carefully, with better timing and a simultaneous opportunity to gain insight into the nature of his emotions and behavior. The therapeutic community will give the patient a chance to strengthen his ego, and integrate better with his follow men. It will enable him to become more mature and better than he ever was, not merely as well. It will permit the patient to act, and sometimes to act-out, not merely be acted upon—to react, rather than just rebel. At the same time the carefully constructed and studied therapeutic community will permit newer and more balanced research into the origins and treatment of mental illness, into the nature of the family, and into the social determinants that affect emotions, attitudes and behavior.

Each institution has an environment, is a milieu in which the patient resides and interacts. In it he may remain the same, get worse or make progress. While much of what happens may be completely outside the control of the hospital treating the patient, a good deal that does happen depends on the nature of the milieu prevailing within the institution.

The aim of every hospital should be to establish a milieu which is therapeutic. However, it has yet to be determined what elements within and about an environment may be considered therapeutic. Certainly an effective drug or an hour of psychotherapy may be considered therapeutic, but it is not this we mean when we speak of the therapeutic community. The fact that therapy is done within the walls of an institution does not necessarily make it a therapeutic community.

During the past seven years we have been attempting to establish a therapeutic community at High Point Hospital. We started basically with the idea that psychotherapy should have a commanding role in the treatment of patients, and that all other therapies should be regarded as subordinate or adjunctive. We started with an abiding faith in insight therapy. We had few and vague ideas about the therapeutic community. After a couple of years of trial and tribulation, if any idea did dawn upon us it was that there had to be "the soil" in which psychotherapy could be done successfully. This was how we thought of it at first—as the soil. We saw that there had to be not only "organization," but proper organization—there had to be not merely personnel, but the right kind of staff. We saw that the hospital was not brick and stone, but the right people. Further, that the "right people" was not enough unless they were correctly integrated. We saw that without this the best people, the best intentions, psychotherapy, shock treatment, tranquilizing drugs—all could be ineffective or, if effective, not to as satisfactory a degree as one would like.

Soon we were thinking and talking about the "therapeutic atmosphere"—that without this we could not do our work effectively or as easily as we might otherwise. The term itself had appeal, and yet had an intangible quality. We could sense that we were trying to make an effective social setting in which to carry out our treatment program. Slowly we began to see that to an increasing extent the social setting *was* the treatment program. We began to speak of the hospital as a society to which the patient was brought—and we saw that this society had its own laws and social relationships, and that these were not much different from those to which the patient had been exposed on the outside. We began to feel and say that our patients were not removed from society, but to a particular kind of society that helped restore their balance and make them more fit than ever to cope with the society from which they had come. We rejected the idea that the hospital was a haven or retreat, and scouted the idea that a patient would get used to the hospital, like to stay, and never want to return home. We said that living in the hospital could be as painful as living anywhere else, and often was. Incidentally, we have not in seven years seen any patient who remained content to stay indefinitely—and feel that this could not occur in a therapeutic community.

There seemed always to be a flaw to our logic which suggested an error in the conclusions we drew from our experience. Perhaps, after all, the patient only responded because he was removed from his traumatic home environment, and thereby relieved of unbearable pressure. Under such conditions he could and did rebound and recuperate, even under the relatively adverse conditions of the poorest hospital milieu. If such argumentation could begin to pass for fact, then the whole concept of the therapeutic community need not be pursued further. It need not be studied or explored with the idea that it had any special therapeutic value and that essentially, then, a hospital was four walls within which individual therapeutic procedures were employed. If positive results followed, then, they were the results of these measures.

In the face of such thinking we were faced with subjecting our social structure to a scrutiny which would expose its component parts, and general attributes.

There are certain principal aspects of a milieu which one might be tempted to consider as a therapeutic community. These factors are both tangible and intangible, and tend to determine the behavior of the patients living in this milieu. A principal determinant of behavior is the general attitude of a medical staff toward its patients. It may tend to treat the disease within a patient, or tend to treat the patient as a person who has a disease. In the former case it may not give much thought to the patient as an individual, whereas in the latter event it gives primary consideration and respect to the individuality of the person and his particular requirements. The basic organization of a mental institution depends very much on the nature of this basic approach. It may be either immense and herd patients together in large wards without much regard for their individual need, or reconstructed as a small unit in which the emotional and personal requirements of a patient may get close attention and adequate satisfaction. In the latter case, a hospital will group its patients rather uniformly, so that relative harmony exists within the group, and differences may be worked out without too great strain or rupture in human relationship. Under this set of conditions a patient may feel the therapeutic sense of belonging he otherwise would not be able to experience. In this manner too the patient is removed from conditions which are too stressful, in keeping with the original intention of hospitalization, and placed in a setting appropriate to his needs. The organization, further, will permit the patient to enter into and participate with other groups as he progresses without sacrificing these therapeutic advantages.

When one has special regard for the patient as an individual, he inevitably will pay heed to patients as a group. The rights of the group are often no less important than those of the individual. The attitude of responsible figures, therefore, to the group's needs, particularly as it may clash with those of the individual, will also determine behavior in any milieu. Ideally, a group is constructed of patients relatively well-matched, in terms of behavior and general temperament so that they may maintain harmonious relationships, and be able to profit by their social interaction. Under the best of conditions and selections, clashes between the needs of the individual and the group arise. When a healthy respect obtains for both, reason and good judgment may be made to prevail. The individual may learn to accept curtailment of his rights without feeling a sacrifice or blow to his self-esteem, but rather enjoy a feeling of gain and self-approval. The patient's ability to accept proper appraisal and adjudication of problems is in essence an indication of his readiness to sustain good group and family living.

The techniques of forming and sustaining these groups is for the moment less important than the recognition of their significance in the general scheme of a therapeutic community, and their function in determining behavior. It should be understood too that these two factors so far mentioned influence the behavior of staff as well as of patients in the milieu in which they all interact.

The team approach to the treatment of patients is a significant positive factor in any therapeutic milieu and favorably determines the behavior of patients. Essentially, the team approach recognizes that all working personnel are important in a true treatment program. Generally the professional members of a staff will arrogate to themselves the entire credit for the therapeutic accomplishments. In some instances, the medical staff will consider sharing this role with the nursing and, perhaps, allied professional departments. This, despite its utter helplessness without efficient and devoted members in every other department which goes to constitute an institution. When personnel generally feel that the better they play their role the better chance the patients have to recover, the better is the therapeutic atmosphere of a hospital community. The spirit which prevails conveys itself to patients, and they enjoy a more wholesome relationship to the non-patients about them. Personnel may have the added satisfaction of knowing that a job well done contributes a helping hand to an ill person.

When a psychotherapeutic program is pursued, the doctor-patient relationship is perhaps the most significant aspect of a therapeutic community. This may be said with full recognition of the fact that it may be useless without other essential factors. Naturally, the nature of this relationship, and the role a physician plays in it are of paramount importance in determining the patient's behavior. Patients will not react uniformly merely because a doctor-patient relationship exists, even in a program devoted to psychotherapy. In a therapeutic community it seems desirable that the psychiatrist play a combined therapeutic and administrative role. Our own experience is that this approach can be highly successful, though extremely difficult. It may prove to be the essence of an ideal therapeutic community. The discussion of this factor alone, and the techniques enabling the therapist to fulfill this role could make several papers in itself. Time limitations, however, will permit me to say no more about it.

The place of value judgments is important in a therapeutic community. Their presence and the exercise of them by the medical staff, or their absence, will have much to do with the behavior of the patients. It is difficult to conceive of a social setting in which value judgments have no place. However, many psychiatrists, particularly psychoanalysts, do not feel they may exercise them in treatment. We, on the other hand, have found that the recognition of the presence of value judgments and their role in determining the attitudes and response of patients, and the conscious application of them in treatment will exert a major positive influence on the progress and behavior of patients. When this is not so, gross as well as subtle acting-out is the rule, and a therapeutic community is most difficult to establish.

The social structure of a community devoted to the care of the mentally ill has much to do with the behavior of its patients. Task-oriented organizations may have any of a variety of structures, and their problems in social relationships develop as functions of these structures. It would be impossible to say which type of structure makes the ideal milieu for a therapeutic community. It is possible that some day one might. In our own case, where we believe we have a therapeutic community, there is a structure which approximates that described as "simple differentiated subordination." There is one person, the Medical Director, responsible for overall control, in whom is vested almost sole authority. The task of treating the patients, however, is divided into parts, and each part is in the hands of a different person, each of whom is responsible to the Medical Director. Thus, there is a Medical, Nursing, Kitchen, Housekeeping, Maintenance, Secretarial and Business Department. Each carries out its own function under a departmental head and there is as little overlapping as possible.

The patient body is small, 35 to 40 patients, and they are housed in one building, so that there is very close proximity between them, and frequent contact amongst themselves and between them and the entire staff. The medical staff is composed of seven full time psychiatrists, and the nursing staff of twenty-one nurses and attendants. Non-professional departments are also highly staffed. Each patient receives a minimum of three therapeutic hours per week, and a great deal of individualized and personalized attention.

In a setting such as I have described a great degree of intimacy develops, and this element would seem to be an ingredient important to a therapeutic community. There is a close "living together" which permits both the healthiest and sickest in an individual to show itself. The intimacy of the entire group permits the therapist to see the patients in action as well as to get first hand reports from all personnel. He need not depend only on the patient's report of himself in psychotherapeutic sessions. At the same time, the patient's irrational reactions are under constant study with him, so that he may gain increasing insight, not merely about his past history and relationships but about his current activities. He may immediately see how his problems hinder his living in the group, and put his new insights to immediate use toward the end of improving his ability to relate in a healthy fashion. Both he and his therapist can see in vivo how he repeats the same sick behavior he did at home. Except that at this time the father and mother, or sister and brother, so conveniently blamed previously, are not present. Instead there are the surrogate figures who are less emotionally involved with him, and therefore capable of helping him understand and change for the better.

Thus, the more closely the milieu provides an atmosphere

which approximates real "living together," the more closely do we approach the concept of the therapeutic community. Such a community would seem to be one that does not merely permit the patient to return to his "normal" prepsychotic state, but really helps him to mature and become a better integrated person than he ever was.

Particularly central to the difficulties of the schizophrenic patient are his problems with authority. When a central figure of authority, therefore, is in close relationship to him his behavior will be influenced. True, it will be in a negative fashion until insight therapy helps him, but he will also be aided if the milieu itself is sufficiently structured in a therapeutic fashion that it permits him to learn from the various experiences this milieu exposes him to. The point I would make is that in a nontherapeutic community these central problems with authority might otherwise be suppressed, only to reappear after hospitalization, or be aggravated and rendered refractory even to psychotherapy of the most intensive nature.

The role which patients are assigned and permitted in a hospital setting will also determine the nature of their behavior. The type of role they have will help determine whether their community is therapeutic or not. As we have seen, patients may be brought to an institution to be gotten out of society's way, or to be acted upon by one therapeutic procedure or another. They may be given certain activities of an occupational and recreational nature. An essential aspect of this role, however, is the attitude of the assigning authorities. It is common to think of occupational and recreational activities as "therapeutic," and they are commonly considered so, but apparently with the underlying philosophy that they divert the patient's mind from his illness, and that busy fingers are thereby kept out of mischief. It may be considered that this is a more subtle form of acting upon the patient, or manner of keeping him out of harm's way within the hospital community itself. It does not necessarily give him an active and participating role that is at the same time functional, in the sense that it is productive and useful to the proper aim or end of the very environment of which he is a member. It would seem that this activity role, with its underlying philosophy, would have to be an integral part of the hospital community one would consider therapeutic.

Ordinarily, and properly so, the patient is the main focus of the hospital community, and it becomes primarily occupied with him and his care. As it is, patients tend to be self-absorbed, and therapy will be directed to diverting them from this self-absorption. Our problem is how best to accomplish this, and at the same time permit the patient's growth and development as a person. It is likely that we should permit them in an organized fashion to act upon the milieu as well as be acted upon. Perhaps they should be permitted an active voice in their community for it to be considered therapeutic in the fuller sense of the word. Again, time will not permit more than this to be said of what would seem to be a significant behavioral determinant in a therapeutic community.

For a lack of time this paper has given but a sketchy idea of the behavioral determinants in a therapeutic community—and, at that, of but a few of these. In different institutions details will differ, depending on many factors, including size, physical plant, training and background of medical staff and policy makers, nature of patients treated and methods of treatment. With time, however, we should be able to define the common ingredients of the therapeutic community, other details notwithstanding, and substantiate the very concept of the therapeutic community. The concept that a milieu per se is therapeutic perhaps should have to prove itself, rather than be taken for granted, as once the germ theory of disease had to prove itself. I have tried to indicate factors that would seem to be important, and that in a hospital community their presence would suggest a milieu we might consider to be therapeutic. Future studies should help us to be more certain of what factors, or combination of factors, distinguish the therapeutic from the non-therapeutic community.

There are some attributes that in general an institution would seem to want to achieve a therapeutic quality. I would say that the hospital should be relatively small, and have good and frequent communication among and between both its staff and patients. The institution should have great flexibility, and the ability and opportunity to change with conditions and the nature of its patients. Individual behavior and the interaction between individual and group should be under constant study. There should be opportunity for patients to gain insight into themselves and others and to appreciate the needs of the group. A therapeutic community will sometimes permit group needs to supersede those of the individual, without the latter suffering a loss of self-esteem. It will show self-absorption to be self-injurious, and consideration of others in team work to be self-healing. It will teach by its structure that nothing is as important to man as his fellow man. Above all the hospital therapeutic community would have to be under the leadership of psychiatrists conversant with psychodynamics who would promote participating behavior appropriate not merely to the patient's own requirements, but to the environment in which he is residing at the time.

Our society is based on respect for the individual and his rights. However, in treating the mentally sick, society,. with little regard for his individual needs, herds him by the thousands into tremendously large institutions, which are generally short-staffed. This is generally attributed to economic necessity and budgetary problems. Economics may only be society's justification and rationalization for its disregard, if not disrespect for and pessimism about the mentally ill.

This paper, thus far, has said nothing about the neuroleptic drugs. Perhaps this has seemed strange and amiss, but I assure you that it was quite intentional and with forethought on my part. I have tried to indicate several factors which quite certainly influence patients' behavior, and to suggest that there are many others which also do. Therapeutic factors may very well be present in such numbers and combinations within an institution as to render that community therapeutic per se, regardless of what drugs it may or may not use.

It would seem, therefore, that in determining the effectiveness of any medication we must be aware of these factors, and the extent to which they are therapeutic. We must know the degree to which they may facilitate the effectiveness of any drug or be the factors which are essentially causing the improvement in patients which we are attributing to the medications. Knowing them we may be able to apply them so much more ably as to make the drugs we know much more effective than they are. If we should gain this greater ability, perhaps we will cease finding ourselves discarding drugs and procedures we have once welcomed with such enthusiasm, only to abandon as having as mysteriously failed us as they once seemed to help us. Such a train of events is neither healthy for psychiatry nor for the public which looks to us for rescue from its malignant malady.

Psychiatrists, as any human beings, will grasp for straws. With the introduction of insulin shock therapy, reports of 90 to 95% cures appeared, and we were carried away with enthusiasm. Thousands of papers were written on the subject, and physiological explanations for its effectiveness were propounded. Yet where is insulin therapy today? Who can report such cures now? That which was once heralded is hardly used today, only some decades since its introduction. Electroshock treatment is not faring much differently. It is not uncommon to hear psychiatrists, who only recently waxed enthusiastic about this procedure, indicate equal enthusiasm about the tranquilizers. They are turning away from shock treatment. The explanations for its effectiveness are no longer meaningful, but those for the new drugs gain credence. How long before we witness the same thing occurring with the tranquilizers which are currently capturing the scene? In the light of what has happened with the others it would not seem far-fetched to forecast the same doom for these drugs in psychiatry.

This is not meant to be a diatribe against the use of physiological procedures and medications. Nor is it meant to indicate that mental illness is not organic in origin nor responsive to physical treatment. The above is called to attention as an historical note. I believe there has been much wasted energy in the way we have treated insulin therapy, and that much of value has been discarded with its abandonment. The same threat exists with regard to electroshock treatment. And unless we approach the study of the new drugs and the determination of their effectiveness differently we may anticipate the same shameful waste of energy. Disappointment will follow disappointment.

Somewhere along the line, and now is as good a time as any—we must stop to assess what we are doing with new methods of treatment. We must subject them to more thorough search and study. Our research approach to them must be multi-dimensional from the start. The cause of mental illness is not simple. Neither are the factors which continue it in motion. Certainly its cure will not be uncomplicated or unidimensional. Conferences such as this should set us on the right track.

7

Role of the Patient in the Therapeutic Community: Patient Participation

ALEXANDER GRALNICK, M.D.
FRANK G. D'ELIA, M.D.

INTRODUCTION

In recent years we have striven in psychiatry not merely to improve specific treatment but to improve and refine our general approach to the patient as a human being. This has been true particularly in the area of hospital care as evidenced by the day-hospital, night-hospital, and open-door policy in the full-time institution. These innovations have been accompanied by efforts to increase both the quantity and quality of hospital personnel, by improving employee practices, and by instituting courses to raise the level of understanding of those directly involved in the treatment of patients. As we have veered from treating the disease within an individual toward consideration of the total person who happens to be ill, we have become more cognizant of him as such, and have tended to attribute to him and to actually give him a more significant role in his treatment program. It is logical, therefore, to study this new role to understand how, if at all, it promotes improvement, and how we may increasingly refine this role.

With the expanding emphasis on the human being it has

Read at the American Psychiatric Association's Southern Divisional Meeting, December, 1958. Reprinted from *American Journal of Psychotherapy,* Vol. XV, No. 1, pp. 63-72. January, 1961.

become quite customary to think of the impact of non-professional as well as professional people on the patient. Thus, what the doctor knows as a physician and prescribes as such is alone not significant; what he is like as a person and how he relates to the patient is equally important. With the growing emphasis on the group of human beings who treat patients, it has been inevitable to think of them all together —personnel and patients—as a community of individuals engaged in a common endeavor, namely, the patient's therapy. The idea of the "therapeutic community" therefore is a natural.

Psychiatrists, eventually, will study the role of each group of participants in the therapeutic process as they are encompassed by the concept. In this paper we will direct our attention to the patients—as individuals and groups of persons in the therapeutic community. First, it is necessary to say a few words about the therapeutic community we call High Point Hospital, within which our patients play the role we are about to discuss. It is a psychiatric facility, housing an average of 40 patients on extensive estate grounds, which devotes itself to an intensive psychoanalytically-oriented program of psychotherapy. Each patient enters voluntarily, and receives three to five treatment sessions weekly in addition to a great deal of individualized management. Physiologic therapies are used, but only adjunctively. Organic cases are excluded and women make up 60 to 70 per cent of the population. Most of the patients are in the range of schizophrenic illness from the most benign or borderline type to those in the acute or chronic stages. There is a sprinkling of patients in other categories, including psychoneuroses and middle-life depressions.

The hospital is accredited for training and has seven full-time therapists, in addition to several supervising and consulting psychiatrists all of whom are analytically trained. In a word, one could describe the atmosphere as that of an active treatment and training center. One large building houses all the patients and is the scene of all indoor activities.

Patients of both sexes reside in close proximity and commingle in routine activities. Accordingly, the therapist may easily observe the gross behavioral patterns of his and other patients, or have them reported to him in conferences by nurses and colleagues who also directly observe this behavior. In addition, of course, he has frequent contact with his patient in sessions where he may observe and hear the patient's emotional reactions to the very incidents the therapist has witnessed himself or had reported to him by others.

As a result of these and other factors there is a rather highly organized therapeutic structure, and administrative procedures and policies evolve from a mass of knowledge derived from this complex of cross references. As a matter of fact, it is for this reason that little distinction is made at High Point between the administrative and therapeutic components of the program; they are considered as two sides of the same coin. Of considerable importance is the fact that much time is regularly spent by the therapist with significant family members. This practice also helps to correlate information and impressions in a first-hand manner. This aspect of our program is maintained by excluding psychiatric social workers, and by gearing the program so that the therapists have sufficient leisure to see the patient's relatives even more often than these ancillary workers ordinarily do. Relatives are also seen by senior staff members who supervise therapy.

The patient population is divided into four groups, in keeping with their level of behavioral integration rather than diagnosis. Each group has a different routine and course of activities, depending on its ability to respect privileges and tolerate responsibilities and social interactivity. Patients tend to move from the restricted group (I) to which they are first assigned when admitted, to the advanced which is an open-floor group with full privileges. For instance, the more restricted, or Group I patients, are semi-disturbed or suicidal and therefore maintained rather exclusively on the closed floor. As improvement occurs they are moved forward by medical conference recommendation into the variety of communal activities usual in psychiatric institutions. Supervision by nursing personnel diminishes as the patient progresses through the intervening groups. In Group IV finally, he may go about the building and grounds more or less as he pleases, but is required to participate in a minimum of group activities at assigned times and to assume some of the community responsibilities which will be described later. This group of patients may visit at home, take educational courses off grounds, and maintain employment in preparation for their eventual departure.

THE PROBLEM

In early 1957 after six years of operation, we considered High Point Hispital a rather highly organized and structured institution but sufficiently flexible and dynamic to be regarded as a therapeutic community—or at least a potential one. However, at the same time, the medical staff had a rather uneasy feeling that something was amiss, as it sensed a certain looseness and purposelessness in its Group IV patients. It observed two things: One, that patients strove to get from Group III, with its relatively structured program, into Group IV, motivated by the idea that they would separate from the group aspects of the program and embark on a course of highly individualistic behavior. This indeed severed them from the cohesive stream of things, which seemed characteristic of the pattern of their illness. At any rate, if this was not their motive, it certainly was the end-result. And this was the second thing observed.

In taking stock of ourselves, the staff could see that its notions of Group IV were perhaps not much different from the patients'. Essentially it was a "free" group. While the group was "required" to eat at certain times and attend occupational therapy at prescribed hours, the group members had "freedom of choice." If they chose not to attend these functions, or to do other things so that they were disruptively late, they felt above criticism. They might find plausible opportunities to be out of the hospital more days than they were in it. We soon found that either the patient in this group divorced himself from the program so completely that he and his family thought it "logical" for him to leave, and this would occur prematurely, or he would "busy" himself about the hospital in a rather isolated manner. No one could find fault with his behavior, but somehow he was no longer in the stream of community activity.

While our program had all the usual earmarks of group and individual activity, we detected a certain passivity about the patients, perhaps what might be termed a lack of community spirit. At times we thought that the patients' main objective in the hospital was merely to get out. Achieving a stable state of mental health seemed to be incidental. If this were so, it would be consistent with prevalent attitudes in society, namely that the psychiatric hospital is the last place to see and the first to flee. At any rate, it seemed that many patients were "waiting" to get well or to be "made" well, and this seemed quite inconsistent with our intensive treatment program and "therapeutic atmosphere." Certainly then, we had to look to ourselves as psychotherapists to solve this situation.

MEETING THE PROBLEM

Accordingly, we started a series of weekly staff conferences to grapple with this problem. Our "most advanced" group seemed a loose collection of individuals who went their separate ways, feeling no group spirit or identity, and existing as a group in name only. Being in this advanced group gave a feeling of "status," but without substance, and allowed "freedom." However, its members "gave" nothing to this group as such, and gained no feeling of pride from its achievements. As we continued to discuss the question, we found we were really searching our own souls and inquiring into our own philosophies of life and moral values. Since the hospital was a small society, what were to be its laws and traditions? Since it was a community in which patients lived rather closely for relatively long periods, did they not owe the group something, even if at some sacrifice? Would they not be healthier if they had a "community feeling"? Should not patients be willing to become more active? Would they not get a feeling of satisfaction and self-esteem from doing something for this "home" in which they lived with fellow patients? Could we accept as "healthy" the attitude of some patients that since this was a private hospital in which they paid for services, they needn't do anything for it? Were they "right"—or healthy—if they could not see that in doing something for the group, they themselves, and not "the hospital," had something to learn and gain? Was a patient "well" if he showed resentment toward the hospital by defacing and neglecting community rooms shared by other patients? Or was this rather a sign of sick disrespect for others?

Soon we found ourselves exploring the concept of "individual freedom" versus "responsibility to the group." Should, or could the sacrifice of an individual desire in the service of the group's need be anything but trauma? Could this on the other hand give a measure of satisfaction and raise one's self-esteem? Was discussion of this nature germane to the subject of treating the psychotic, particularly the schizophrenic? Some of us thought our questions were pertinent because we were observing the patient's socially pathologic behavior in the community setting. If they were to go uninfluenced, then we would have a pathologic community—not a therapeutic one. What steps, then, were we to take which would establish a more thorough therapeutic community in the midst of all this individually and socially pathologic behavior so they could be more effectively controlled and channelled into healthier avenues?

As our conferences progressed, we came to certain conclusions and took concrete steps. Essentially our problem was to weld this group of patients into a unit, to make them "feel" as a group and identify with it. We knew this would have to be done against their own pressures to fragment and to seek isolated positions (to avoid social integration because of their personal preoccupations). Toward this end we introduced some new rules which would require their attendance at certain functions so that they could in fact meet as a group. These included meals, occupational therapy activities, and social affairs. In addition, the allotted time permitted out of the hospital was reasonably curtailed. We believed that the more consistent application of precepts in itself would promote a stronger group feeling.

Our most significant decision was that of establishing regular meetings of these patients under the guidance of one of our therapists. As the medical conferences had progressed, the patients had been given in their individual sessions some idea of our proceedings, waited with bated breath for their outcome, and at the same time made some of their ideas known to us. The thought of "group meetings" took hold, particularly since their ideas "as a group" would be sought. It was explained that simultaneously we wished to convey our ideas as a medical group to them. Our first plan for their consideration was the establishment of several patient committees to participate in community hospital activities.

These group meetings have continued to the present time, but the most stimulating ones occurred in the first few months when the patients planned with us the program which finally evolved. The staff member who presided at these meetings reported their tenor to the medical staff. The staff, in turn, gave guidance to him and had him convey our reactions and further suggestions to the patients. Naturally the pathologic behavior of individual patients came out in such a meeting, and eventually was channeled to their therapists to be worked out in therapy. The pressure on the part of staff and patients to convert these meetings into group therapy sessions was combatted. However, the meetings were tape-recorded so therapists could hear them, and the reactions of the patients were discussed freely at our staff meetings. Sometimes therapists could be instructed to work out specific problems with their patients on the strength of the patients' reactions in these group meetings.

Space does not permit me to relate even a part of the rich discussion which followed, nor to recount exactly the steps in the evolution of this aspect of the patient's role in our therapeutic community. Suffice it to say that spirited conferences ensued. Essentially, the staff conveyed the concept that the patients were a social group living in a small society to which they should have real ties. Our belief was that they had much to gain by doing things for the group with which they lived. In this manner we drew a parallel between the patients as a group and a family situation. The members of a family could go their separate ways, or work cooperatively for the common good and gain a healthy satisfaction thereby.

It was interesting to see how the patients divided into two camps, one thinking that only "the hospital" would gain, and the other that the patients themselves had everything to gain. The one group tallied the amount of dollars the hospital would save by their labors and devised methods for their compensation, while the other group spoke in terms of the greater good—something which could not be measured in terms of dollars. The one group found fault with most suggestions and delayed implementation of ideas, whereas the other enthusiastically developed the program. Particularly with reference to housekeeping activities, the males in the negative group objected because this was "a woman's work, not man's." Thus, this common problem of the division of labor by sex showed itself here too.

THE "PRODUCTIVE DAY"

The idea of "the productive day" was introduced, and implemented by the formation of several committees. The aim was not activity just for its own sake or for individual diversion, but for the positive effect on the patient from such participation in the useful work which fulfilled the needs of the group. If they worked together it was expected, too, that the ties among patients would be strengthened. It was recognized, of course, that the emotional problems each had in relating to others would be highlighted. Naturally, these problems would then be worked through in individual therapy. The problems of the group, as such, would be handled through its contact with the medical staff as a group.

At about this time, as fate would have it, the hospital's housekeeping department suffered serious losses. The staff decided to ask the Group IV patients if they would help out by assuming the housecleaning of their open floor. They thrashed this out in their group meeting as indicated above. Soon a housekeeping committee was set up with a chairman and membership which had assigned tasks. Ultimately, too, the male patients were involved in this work. This committee, now including patients of still another group, continues to function to this day, and manages practically all of the housekeeping of its floor.

Consonant with the concept of involving patients in useful community tasks, other patient committees were organized by mutual consent of the staff and patients. These include the library, garden and grounds, newspaper, and entertainment committees. In addition, patients undertake individual assignments, such as occupational therapy, assisting in the dining-room, and group tasks of a non-recurring nature. Space limitations do not permit a detailed description of these committees and their work. However, they all function—their efficiency, of course, depending on the individual patients of which they are composed. For instance, the patients publish a newspaper every six weeks or so, gathering contributions from all groups of patients; they plan a weekly party or cook-out, help to make drapes, plan gardens, and conduct games for the closed-floor patients.

COMPLEXITIES OF THE PROGRAM

A program of this nature can be quite complex and can give rise to many complications. It requires constant vigilance on the part of the medical and nursing staff, and the understanding by all that final decisions and judgments always lie in the hands of the medical staff. Although the patients are active participants in the planning and execution of projects, they must understand that the therapeutic staff is the final arbiter. The staff, on the other hand, must be flexible and mindful of the therapeutic aspects and implications for the patients of the program's every detail. Accordingly, it must be realistic, though not arbitrary, and ready to risk accepting certain suggested plans which may not succeed. The gain for the patients of such an expression of faith may outweigh the ensuing difficulties, and offer them an opportunity to learn by their errors. In addition, they stand to profit from the demonstrated give-and-take when they and the staff, as groups of individuals, are in disagreement. As significant as anything is the opportunity the patients have to deal with figures of authority who prove to be hardly as unreasonable, awesome, and overpowering as they had always imagined such people to be. Schizophrenics, particularly, have marked problems with symbols of authority, and the chance to relate to them in this living situation is especially valuable therapeutically.

This kind of a program requires the medical staff to exercise greater care than ever before in advancing a patient to Group IV. The patient must be sufficiently stable and intact to participate in its program. Otherwise he may become a disruptive force. On the other hand, the nature of this group and its plan offers the patient entering it an opportunity to integrate on a healthier level, and test himself in task-situations similar to those he will soon meet at home. We have developed certain techniques to effectuate a smoother and successful graduation into Group IV. Success is important to save the patient the trauma of failure in his group. When a patient is considered for Group IV, the staff must feel convinced that he understands and is willing to participate in its program. The patient is then required to attend meetings of the group as a test of his reactions, and to aid him to decide if he is ready. If he is, he and his therapist then prepare a program of activities which involve the patient in various committees. An attempt is made to strike a fair balance between the time given to group work, individual projects, and leisure.

RESULTING CHANGES

The changes which occurred in the hospital subsequent to this new program's introduction cannot be detailed here. The overall difference was commonly described as a "change in morale." The general attitude of the patients toward the hospital became much more wholesome. Carping about relatively minor things markedly diminished and the common complaint that the hospital was only interested in "making money" also subsided to a surprising degree. Some patients actually offered contributions to the institution. Patients reported a change in their attitude toward nursing personnel with whom they now worked on projects. They felt their contact with employees to be broadened beyond that of patient-nurse. We felt that there was an air of greater activity about getting well, rather than the passivity which we had sensed before. Patients no longer sought entrance to Group IV to achieve "freedom to do as one pleased" but to forward their state of health. There seemed to be a feeling of more cohesiveness about the Group IV patients, and a freer expression of initiative on their part. These patients seemed to become more interested in the welfare of the lower group patients, and showed a willingness to help them. The hospital as an organization began to take on a stability and solidity it had appeared to lack. Individualizing the program of patients also seemed to become easier.

Significantly, a wholesome change occurred in the general

attitude toward authority. Ordinarily, the patients' problems in this area had been demonstrated by the covert and overt expression of hostility toward the Director. This had become a more or less accepted phenomenon since he was a central figure of authority and it was common for patients, either as individuals or as groups, to blame him for mishaps or disappointments which befell them in the hospital. This attitude showed a marked change for the better with the change in program. It was something he could feel, and others of the staff could confirm, both from their general observations and from individual sessions with patients. This "happier" relationship between the patients and Director has continued to the present.

PREREQUISITES AND PRINCIPLES

There are undoubtedly various ways in which the patient may participate in a particular therapeutic community. The nature of his role, however, will depend on several factors, including his caliber, level of integration, and ability. The success of any program similar to that outlined above will depend on such prerequisites as the presence of long-term patients, the quantity and quality of personnel, size of patient population, stability of employment among professional personnel, proper organization of non-professional departments and the flexibility of the psychiatric staff as authority figures.

Certain principles act as guides in developing such a therapeutic role for patients. The careful structuring of the program by the medical staff is essential. Behavior and the evolution of healthy activity are seen as influenced by the nature of the program established. Feelings and attitudes are considered to be affected, if not determined, by the nature of behavior, as well as the traditions, mores, and moral values of the hospital community. Inasmuch as the psychiatric hospital is a society of groups, as well as individuals, it must have formulated customs. Principal among these should be the belief that the expression of individual freedom is to be tempered by the needs of the group.

SUMMARY

This paper relates the need for and the development of a patient-participation program in an in-patient setting. Its role and effect in a particular type of therapeutic community is described, as is the therapeutic milieu itself. Complexities, prerequisites, and principles for the establishment of such a program are outlined.

8

The Therapeutic Community as an Insight Catalyst: Expanding the Transferential Field

EDWIN L. RABINER, M.D.
EFRAIN GOMEZ, M.D.
ALEXANDER GRALNICK, M.D.

THE RIGOROUS APPLICATION of the scientific method to the elevation of treatment parameters has clearly demonstrated the vital role played by the total context in which a treatment is given. Field factors may act synergistically with or antagonistically against the treatment agent itself. They may vitiate the effectiveness of a potent treatment agent or create the illusion that an inert agent is effective. It therefore comes as no surprise that the Expert Committee on Mental Health of the World Health Organization concluded in a recent report that "the most important single factor in the efficacy of the treatment given in a mental hospital appears to be an intangible element that can only be described as atmosphere."

The study, manipulation, and control of factors determining the "atmosphere" has in recent years become a high-ranking order of business for the hospital psychiatrist. He has been challenged to leave the security of the one-to-one doctor-patient relationship and to expand his role beyond

Reprinted from *American Journal of Psychotherapy,* Vol. XVIII, No. 2, pp. 244-258. April, 1964.

that of directly administering a treatment agent to the patient, be it drug, shock, psychotherapy, or any combination of the three.

Advancing knowledge has defined for him the task of programmatically applying his understanding of the determinants of mental health and pathology to the planning and manipulation of the residential treatment center's social structure, value systems, and transactional models,[1,2] for these are the factors that determine "atmosphere."

The burgeoning literature on the "Therapeutic Community" attests to our growing involvement in the study and therapeutic utilization of the "total treatment field." A plethora of concepts has been advanced as guidelines for the transformation of wards and hospitals into therapeutic communities.[3-9] These include: opening channels of communication, broadening the traditional decision-making process to include all participants in unit life, the firm expectation of socially acceptable behavior, increasing interaction, emphasis on group process, opening doors, giving patients increasing responsibility for the direction of their daily activities, substituting an interested and helpful peer group for tangible authority against whom the patient can react and rationalize, supplanting excessive imposed controls, restrictions, regimentation and tradition-bound rituals with self-control, dignity, and trust.

Making explicit the way in which such concepts and procedures act to ameliorate psychopathology and integrating them within the psychodynamic frame of reference with which we are accustomed to conceptualize psychopathology is no easy task. To date, despite the prolific enthusiasm of the advocates of "The Therapeutic Community," we are far from conceptual, no less, implementational closure. Rather, one is left with the feeling that exposure to a certain kind of milieu or social field can in some implicit and perhaps even "magic fashion" be expected to have a therapeutic effect on disturbed functioning. The difficulty of explicitly integrating psychodynamic concepts and social processes has led many to feel, "It's fine to open channels of communication and bring democratic process to the ward, but what has this to do with 'cure'? The important treatment of the patient goes on in my office!" The response of others[10] has been that the therapeutic community "fosters a transference cure rather than one gained through insight which may be less stable than one gained through personal growth."

There are many[11,12] in the ranks of those who have witnessed first-hand reconstructive therapeutic change evolve from patient participation in medically planned social process who would vigorously protest such a downgrading of results they have observed. These workers, and we number ourselves among them, would question the implication that the result is inferior simply because the process of change has yet to be explicitly stated in the more familiar terms of the individual psychodynamic frame of reference. If, however, we are to expect our more traditionally oriented colleagues to accompany us on the journey into the promising reaches of psychosocial exploration, it is incumbent upon us to attempt to translate our experience and observations from the interactional to the psychodynamic framework. In this report we hope to make explicit one area of convergence of these two conceptual systems.

THE THERAPEUTIC COMMUNITY AS A TRANSFERENTIAL VANTAGE POINT

It is generally accepted that dreams, free associations, and transference phenomena comprise the windows through which we may view the unconscious and reconstruct the patient's significant past. Because psychiatric inpatients so often will not or cannot comply with "The Fundamental Rule," we are likely in our treatment of them to be denied all save the last of these vantage points—the transference. This is particularly true where reality testing is impaired to the point that demands for spurious transference gratifications or fear and distrust of others prevent an adequate perception of the true nature and purpose of the psychotherapeutic relationship. In such instances, the communication level essential to traditional forms of self-inquiry can seldom be achieved.

Many therapists have spent years patiently gratifying transference demands or assuming a consistently empathic, nonjudgmental, and permissive posture vis à vis the patient, or both, in the hope of overcoming this initial obstacle to treatment. The financial considerations involved in intensive psychoanalytically oriented inpatient care, let alone the price the patient pays in terms of prolonged removal from the extramural stream of life, have led to the search for new techniques to expedite therapeutic engagement.

In our own efforts toward this end we have attempted to make maximal use of the transferential vantage point which, of the three enumerated data sources, is least dependent upon the patient's conscious cooperation. We have sought to do so through (a) planned efforts to promote the crystallization of multiple transferences onto others in the inpatient social field, and (b) a painstakingly maintained observational and communication matrix designed to promptly funnel to the individual therapist accurate observations of his patient's transferential behavior.

A STRUCTURAL MODEL FOR EXPANDING THE TRANSFERENTIAL FIELD

To achieve this objective we have established an operational model within our 40-bed psychoanalytically oriented treatment setting which has been described more fully elsewhere.[9] In addition to strategic placement with roommates and tablemates, patients are assigned to activity groups designed to hold them in a fixed social context within which transferential behavior can develop, be observed, and dealt with in individual psychotherapy. Each activity group reflects a level of demand for adequate interpersonal behavior, the levels ranging from parallel or simply contiguous to rather complex, cooperative task-oriented activity. The individual patient is placed in specific social contexts whose demands are both commensurate with his response capacities and appropriate to the intermediary goals of his psychotherapy. He remains in these contexts until such time as emerging transferential behavior in relation to them has been brought to awareness and worked through. When the psychotherapeutic yield reaches the point of diminishing returns, he is reassigned, generally proceeding in sequence from the lesser to the more demanding social context.

As the behavioral expression of active psychopathology comes under sufficient control to permit reasonably effective participation in cooperative task-oriented activity, patients are assigned to one or several patient committees. There are six such committees, appointed by the Medical Staff and supervised by a resident therapist, comprising the patient participation program. Each of these assumes responsibility for the execution and further elaboration of a set of services to the hospital community. The Library Committee, for example, selects and purchases new books and periodicals, distributes books to sicker patients, catalogues volumes in the patient and hospital medical libraries, plans and leads weekly discussion groups and musicales. Committee tasks range from menial to creative, and require relatedness to objects, skills and people. Individual roles include follower, collaborator, planner, and leader. Our therapists, in serving as advisors to one or more committees, observe the behavior of their own and other patients in this task-oriented interpersonal context, arbitrating differences between committee and medical staff. Within this format a wide range of functional capacities and interpersonal patterns can be scrutinized, experimented with, and tested. Specific aberrant attitudes can be exposed and worked through along the lines described by Saslow and Meterazzo.[13]

This model has enabled us to escape the temporal limits of the three to five psychotherapeutic interviews per week and to utilize the patient's total waking experience in the hospital to carry forward our inquiry into the nature of his difficulties. Therapist and patient alike are, in a manner of speaking, thus able to watch in the unfolding multiple transferences a documentary film on the significant occurrences in the patient's life and his reactions and adaptation to them.

Where work with the irrational elements characterizing the patient's interpersonal transactions within the hospital has progressed sufficiently, and wherever it is feasible, members of the biologic family are added to the observational field via the inauguration of conjoint family interviews. In this higher life proximity situation transferential behavior is further scrutinized and therapeutic gains are tested along lines described in a previous report.[14] The application of this approach is illustrated below.

CASE MATERIAL

A. *History*

Gwen, a 22-year old white divorcee, was admitted to the hospital in August, 1960 with a diagnosis of Chronic Undifferentiated Schizophrenic Reaction with sociopathic features. Her history revealed a long-standing life-pattern disorganization punctuated in recent years by episodes of alcoholism, erratic behavior, extremely poor judgment, and promiscuity. These episodes had followed a divorce from her husband, an alcoholic who had treated her sadistically, beating her, and demanding her collaboration in perverse sexual behavior. Gwen had passively submitted to her husband's abusiveness and then to her father's uninvited dissolution of the marriage.

Gwen was the older by two years of two daughters born to the first marriage of her father, an affluent business executive. Her parents had separated when she was eight years old, and the mother took the children to California. She died three years later of a self-administered overdose of barbiturates. Gwen remembered her mother as very strict and distant. She had devoted herself to the Bahai religion "in order to give up drinking. She died in her sleep." Gwen was happy to return to her father and dismayed at his remarriage six months later to a woman Gwen described as "controlling and overwhelming." Gwen was jealous of her sister whom she saw as the father's favorite. Her father and stepmother described the sister as the more stable of the two. She made a satisfactory marriage and has been residing with her husband in Utah.

Gwen's school performance had been very poor. She attributed this to a lack of confidence in herself and recalled feeling in school like "the ugly duckling." Although her father had used his influence to secure a college acceptance for Gwen, she had sabotaged her father's efforts by marrying an uneducated bartender over vigorous parental opposition. The marriage ended in divorce after one year during which she had been unfaithful on numerous occasions.

B. *Mental Status*

At the time of her admission to our closed ward, Gwen was three months pregnant out of wedlock. Psychiatric examination revealed a very pretty, well-dressed young woman whose manner was passive but pleasant and ingratiating. Her affect was constricted at a moderately depressed level. Although grossly her thought processes appeared relatively intact, examination elicited evidence of autistic and symbolic thinking. With much prodding she stated her plans for the future in the following rather pathetic and very empty fashion: "I guess I'll stay here until the baby comes and then do whatever my family wants." A few weeks after admission, she had a spontaneous and uneventful abortion to which she appeared quite indifferent.

C. *Course in the Hospital*

This was the sum and substance of our knowledge of Gwen and her problems at the outset of her treatment. Efforts made during ensuing weeks to get more detailed information from the family ran afoul of their aloofness, feelings of "good riddance," and the father's direct refusal to discuss his first marriage or anything related to it. Used to commanding and buying compliance, the father made it clear that he did not wish to be bothered. The stepmother saw Gwen as a bad girl and a disgrace to the family whose reputation and good appearance had to be maintained at all costs.

In psychotherapeutic interviews, Gwen appeared confused, anergic, and without any sense of self or hope for her future. She volunteered nothing and responded to direct questions in a scanty and evasive manner. Her stated self-concept was that of a stupid and uninteresting young woman and she appeared defeated and resigned to her fate. On the ward she was compliant, responding pleasantly when approached but generally taking little initiative and remaining uninvolved with others. Thus over the first two months direct efforts to explore with the patient or her family the experential determinants of her difficulties were unavailing.

Although Gwen showed no interest in the matter, she was moved to the open floor. This was done in the hope that exposure to better integrated, more socially responsive patients would foster greater involvement by virtue of which a template of her neurosis would be crystallized onto the hospital's social field. Gwen promptly ran into two kinds of difficulty. She became frightened of a middle-aged, domineering roommate who treated her as though she were a servant. Although her enslavement to this woman was known to the staff, "Cinderella" said nothing of it to her therapist, who was soon to become "Prince Charming." A second area of tension developed in relation to other female patients of her therapist as Gwen began to resent any attention paid to them.

She remained relatively uncommunicative in her sessions but began to bring in dreams as gifts to her therapist. She would recite the dreams but showed no interest in working with them. Careful comparison of her dream material, with which the therapist was in constant touch via collateral informants, revealed clear-cut point-to-point correlations.

The following examples illustrate the usefulness of such comparisons in expanding one's understanding of the dynamic factors underlying the illness of an uncooperative patient.

1. It had been observed that visits by her stepmother left Gwen extremely distraught, although she said nothing about it to her therapist. He discontinued these visits over her objection that doing so would antagonize her stepmother. Gwen brought her first dream to the next session. "My roommate gave me black pills to take. I was terrified." For the first time she verbalized in association to this dream her fear of her roommate's aggressiveness. "She can see right through me. I have to stare into space to protect myself from her." A second dream reported in the next hour further established the nature of her transference to her roommate. "I got a letter from my mother stating that she couldn't come to visit but instead was sending presents in a plastic bag. I felt frightened." Gwen associated the plastic bag with death. Her mother had "seen through" the discontinuation of her visits, assumed her daughter did not wish to see her and was retaliating under the guise of maternal solicitude.

2. Somewhat later the therapist was advised by the nursing staff that when he made his rounds as duty officer and did not see Gwen first, she would become upset and request sedation. Yet when he entered her room, Gwen would close the door and promptly lapse into an uncommunicative and obviously uncomfortable state. In sessions she refused to acknowledge having any particular feelings toward the therapist. Similarly, she said nothing to him about the fact that another of the therapist's female patients, who felt erotically attracted to him, had begun to needle and criticize her at the dinner table. She did, however, report a dream in which this patient was chasing her with a prayer book. The scene then abruptly shifted to one in which "father was trying to do something to me near an elevator shaft."

3. One day Gwen reacted violently, stomping out of the room when another of her therapist's patients remarked,

"You know, Gwen, we can share him." Gwen, of course, did not speak of this occurrence but the next day reported having dreamt "I was smothering my sister to death." In the absence of Gwen's associations, the meaning of this dream was nevertheless revealed in the nurse's report of the previous day's incident.

Thus from data comprised of the manifest content of these and other dreams along with detailed information about her hospital relationships supplied by others, a dynamic formulation of Gwen's illness began to suggest itself. Incestuous wishes lay at the root of her fearful compliance with the wishes of aggressive women who "could see through me." These wishes were now clearly focused on her therapist, who accordingly asked her, "Is it possible that the dreams and discussions centered about your father are being stimulated by our relationship?"

Gwen at once became mobile and expressive in contrast to her former lifeless impassive posture during interviews. Hesitantly she began to verbalize grandiose, referential ideas about the therapist, believing him to be infatuated with her. She revealed a number of previously unreported dreams about him which made clear her wish for romantic attention from him. To her despair, however, the therapist always eluded her in these dreams. In the ensuing weeks she stubbornly refused to discuss her feelings for the therapist directly. She stopped reporting dreams and said little about her behavior outside the office. The intensity of her wish for absolute possession of him continued, however, to evidence itself in her complaints to others of his coldness and disinterest and her increasingly competitive acting out with his other female patients.

Gwen was in her tenth hospital month when she spontaneously discussed with her therapist the sexual advances being made to her by a psychopathic male patient. At this time the staff had become concerned about her on several scores. She seemed more and more to be isolating herself from her peers and had become extremely seductive toward very sick male patients. In sessions she seemed, if anything, more sullen and remote. Her therapist was aware, however, that her jealousy had been fanned to uncontrollable heights by the fact that he had been forced to spend additional time with a young woman who had become acutely psychotic—a patient who had borrowed Gwen's sweaters and jewelry to wear to sessions with him.

The meaning of Gwen's seductiveness with other men became clear. The therapist interpreted this to Gwen as a replaying both of her vindictive and self-debasing marriage when "sent away" to school by her father, and of her promiscuity when rejected by her husband. Gwen angrily replied, "I don't care what I'm doing. I just do it." When it was learned through another patient that Gwen was about to elope with one of the hospital groundsmen, she was returned for her own protection to the closed floor. In response to repeated confrontations with the determinants of her promiscuous "antisocial behavior," Gwen finally blurted out "You made me love you and now you refuse to go all the way. To hell with you." Gwen's transference neurosis, fanned to a white heat by her dealings with mother and sister surrogates within the hospital had burst with explosive force into the open where she could see it and feel it.

The major therapeutic task was now clear. Having furnished the essential diagnostic information, the milieu could now be utilized in a planned fashion to gratify Gwen's needs, at least in part, while providing opportunity for social relearning. In the security and reduced complexity of the closed floor, with a great deal of attention from her therapist and much deliberately maternal nursing care, Gwen began to emerge from her defensive cocoon. Gradually, tentatively, she began on her own to discuss parallels between her hospital behavior and the prior events of her life and see the oedipal determinants of both. She began to make things in occupational therapy for other female patients. Her dreams confirmed her wishes to get closer to mother and sister surrogates. Yet in these dreams her gifts, tokens of amnesty, would either disappear or be rejected.

She continued during this interval to see herself as stupid and worthless, or else as a sexual object to be used and then discarded. In sessions, she expressed guilt over her previous sexual behavior and a total lack of satisfaction in it. Fellatio performed on her husband had brought greatest satisfaction but, other than via masturbation, she had never achieved orgasm. As this material came up, Gwen began to run indiscriminately to other patients on the ward to be cuddled and held.

The therapist, mustering current experiential reinforcement, was then able to point out that what she seemed to need most desperately, and had actually been seeking in her promiscuous behavior, was a very primitive and essentially maternal kind of warmth, symbolized through fellatio as reunion with the breast. In her dreams during this period, men were represented as objects upon which she urinated, or as birds who would come to her only when she would feed them, again suggesting that her sexual promiscuity was fulfilling primarily pregenital needs. This interpretation was followed by diminished acting out of her oedipal transference and she was moved back to the open floor.

At the end of 16 months of treatment, Gwen had gained considerable insight, was relating quite appropriately to her therapist, and seemed to be working well in therapy. However, what was going on beyond the office was in sharp contrast to her apparent improvement in the one-to-one relationship. For it was reported that she had not been taking medicine that she was to have taken during week-end visits, had been drinking and had dropped out of hospital committee activities without discussing this with her therapist. Evidence came to light that she was having secret encounters with outsiders. In a less flagrant way, she remained committed to punishing the therapist for failing to love her by being a "lost woman."

Now, however, Gwen was able to see more accurately

her own reflection in the hospital's looking glass. Accordingly, she complained to her therapist of being excluded and of feeling like a persona non grata among her fellow patients, for the first time actively seeking his help with a problem. Although many cliques and close friendships had developed within the hospital, the fact was that Gwen was indeed friendless. He reviewed with Gwen the oedipally determined nature of her relationships with women, characterized by fearful compliance alternating with blatant disregard, while she had periodically bought the affection of men with all her energies. The reason for the negative social response to her became immediately clear. The oedipal parallel seemed equally clear. Her predatory attitude toward her father might well have alienated her mother, stepmother, and sister.

Along with this insight, she expressed her determination to work through the rivalrous feelings toward women which underlay her compliance, no matter how much effort it would require. She began tentatively to reach out and to attempt realistic self-assertion, discussing these efforts in detail during therapy sessions. In the hospital community, with the support of the social group worker, whose aid was enlisted by the therapist, she began to experiment with effective assertion. For instance, as a member of the House Committee, she became involved in a power struggle with the housekeeper, a middle-aged, authoritarian woman who reacted with angry condescension to Gwen's efforts at self-assertion. The social group worker mollified and supported the housekeeper, while the therapist supported the appropriateness of Gwen's behavior toward her. She was assigned to the Newspaper Committee where she had to approach female patients for contributions and handled these transactions quite well.

Arrangements were made at her initiative for her to work in the hospital beauty parlor, under the supervision of the hospital beautician, a warm and understanding person, and the social group worker.

At this point, during her sixteenth hospital month, the therapist, for quite understandable reasons, began to pat himself on the back. After all, Gwen's oedipal conflict had been brought to full awareness and abreacted in the transference, following which she had achieved an apparently better level of interpersonal activity. She now seemed to be relating constructively and cooperatively to the "hospital family."

Staff members continued to report, however, that while Gwen displayed apparent enthusiasm for her work in the hospital beauty salon, and seemed to be functioning well in her committee work, they still sensed in her a beaten, lifeless quality which was no longer apparent to her therapist. The director of nursing suggested that this seemed most noticeable after Gwen's return from week-end visits which had been reestablished.

When she was with her own family, her hard-won gains apparently did not stand up. She told the therapist with great despair that her stepmother seemed to resent any attention paid to her by her father and frequently planned social events during Gwen's visits from which she was excluded. Because of the difficulty in determining from Gwen's second-hand reports the relative contributions to this impasse of her own and her family's pathology, it was decided to embark on a series of conjoint family interviews. Gwen's stepmother indicated her willingness to participate but hastened to add that her husband would be unable to attend. Although apprehensive at the prospect, Gwen saw the value of testing her gains in a series of family interviews and agreed to go along with them.

The first few meetings were characterized by a marked lack of spontaneity and considerable tension between Gwen and her stepmother. Finally, her stepmother became annoyed and complained, "What's the point of this. If you have something to say Gwen, say it!" Gwen blurted out that she couldn't because her stepmother could never be understanding. Her stepmother replied, "You're the only one who thinks so." "Oh no, I'm not. Sandy (Gwen's sister) thinks you're a bitch too." In a rage her stepmother said, "I won't put up with this. I'm the one who is holding the family together. Your father's at the breaking point. I'm playing nursemaid to him. Your sister is like you—irresponsible."

Gwen's stepmother failed to keep several subsequent family therapy appointments. When Gwen phoned to inquire about it, her stepmother said, "Go to hell. You can have your father all to yourself." The environmental contribution to Gwen's oedipal bind was clear and irrefutable!

On the premise that the full force of their differences should be aired while Gwen was still in the protective environment of the hospital, the therapist was able to persuade the stepmother to resume the joint interviews. At one of these sessions, the stepmother began to compare her own virtues favorably with those of Gwen's mother, exposing her own rivalrous feelings. For the first time Gwen was told that her mother had disappeared on alcoholic debauches for long periods of time and had been in and out of mental hospitals during Gwen's childhood. In intercurrent individual sessions, the therapist helped Gwen to see in these revelations about her mother the pregenital roots of her own oedipal strivings.

Gwen's stepmother then turned her fury on the father. After roundly criticizing him as a mental case himself, she added that he complained about having to drive Gwen to and from the hospital on visits. Gwen asked, "Why didn't he tell me to my face? Can't he come to these sessions?" The stepmother said, "He had no time and besides he's scared to death of psychiatrists."

Gwen then asserted her wish to remain in the hospital on week ends, secretly hoping her father would visit, telephone, or write. When he failed to do so, she became angry with the therapist and immediately became involved with an immature adolescent patient. This behavior was interpreted in the light of previous, similar episodes of acting out and Gwen immediately grasped the full significance of its meaning, promptly discontinuing the affair.

When the father finally agreed to come to the conjoint sessions, his extreme defensiveness led the therapist to proceed with great caution. This gave Gwen the impression that the therapist had abandoned her. "How can I stand up to them if you can not?" she asked. As the conjoint sessions continued, with the therapist both encouraging her and leading the way himself, Gwen became increasingly assertive. This led to an unsuccessful attempt by the stepmother to sabotage the joint sessions. She instructed her husband to make excuses for her inability to attend and then waited for him in the car outside. In the stepmother's absence, the family's pathology was quickly unmasked. The father sat in the therapist's chair in a gesture of contempt for the therapist. He took over the meetings. At times he ogled Gwen and held her hand while talking down to her. He squashed Gwen's every endeavor at self-assertion. Thus, on one occasion, when Gwen was talking about her future in a reasonable way, her father interrupted her, asking sarcastically, "and then what?" When Gwen replied, "I'll get married to someone decent," her father cruelly responded, "What do you have to offer?"

Thus it became apparent that Gwen's growing independence was threatening to both parents. Her stepmother needed to keep Gwen and her father from each other. Her father needed to maintain Gwen's sick dependence upon him, playing out his game of seduction and rebuff for his own masculine aggrandizement.

Gwen could not see clearly that she had been trapped in an impossibly conflicting and destructive family situation. With the insight gained from the direct witnessing of this dramatic replication, her behavior in the hospital changed dramatically. She became outgoing, spontaneous, and animated. She was elected chairman of the Newspaper and House Committees. (It is interesting to note that her liabilities in these areas had been very marked. She had originally been unable to make her own bed, take care of her room, and had felt too stupid to read the headlines of a newspaper or write an adequate letter.) The psychic energy dissipated in multiple transference attitudes was now available for activity useful to herself and to the community. Others, including the therapist, were perceived and accepted as they really were for the first time in her life.

Plans were now made for Gwen's discharge. The suggestion that she live away from her family met with little resistance, as all parties concerned had seen in the family interviews a graphic demonstration of the pitfalls involved in their living together. She began meetings with the psychiatrist with whom she would be in aftercare, with a vocational counselor, and with a home-finding service and was discharged in March, 1963 as much improved.

Course Following Discharge

Four months have now elapsed since Gwen's discharge. She has found congenial quarters with a family in Manhattan that has several other boarders and has arranged to begin classes in Commercial Art. She has become engaged to a warm, sensitive, and extremely understanding accountant whom she met shortly after leaving the hospital. She visits her family infrequently but maintains regular telephone contact with her stepmother. Her father has been drinking heavily and has been openly philandering. Faced with more formidable rivals for her husband's affections, her stepmother has begun to commiserate with Gwen about her difficulties with him. Gwen has been able to feel a genuine sympathy for her which has enabled her to speak supportively to her mother, avoiding both falling prey to the illusion of reunion with the mother and efforts to satisfy competitive or vindictive needs. She has analytic sessions three times a week, works well with her own dream material, and freely discusses her feelings about the therapist to whom she relates quite appropriately. There has been no recurrence of promiscuity or alcoholic excess. She spends a fair amount of time with women friends, including several friends from the hospital who have been discharged. Within the context of her relationship with her fiancé, traces of her fear of abandonment and displacement remain to be worked through but these are within manageable proportions.

DISCUSSION

We have described a treatment approach to a difficult group of patients which seeks to capitalize on the multileveled observations of transference behavior that can be made in the inpatient setting. Strategic use is made of the variety of bound social contexts that exist or can be built into the therapeutic community for the crystallization of transference attitudes and behavior. Accumulating data in this regard provide a basis for the therapist's intervention on two levels: (a) the interpretive promotion of self-awareness, and (b) the specific prescription of increasing social participation in order to expose more fully pathologic perceptions, attitudes, and behavior and to provide opportunity for social relearning. Not only does the approach described afford a rich source of information for the therapist with respect to individual diagnostic formulation, timing of interpretations, and evaluation of the "working through process," but it provides an impetus for treatment engagement as well, as the patient is confronted in the highly charged present context with the social response appropriate to his or her interpersonal behavior.

We have illustrated the usefulness of this approach with case material highlighting the events in the social, intrapsychic, and family fields which contributed to the patient's deepening insight and emotional growth.

Our patient entered the hospital in a state of utter resignation and withdrawal. Initial efforts by her therapist in the one-to-one psychotherapeutic relationship to interest her in herself and to mobilize her energies for the process of self-inquiry were to no avail. She could not be hatched from her hollow shell of pleasant compliance until she was strategically moved to facilitate transferential developments. Brought then by the force of her erotic transference into conflict with maternal and filial surrogates in the persons of other of her therapist's female patients, Gwen's energies were dramatically turned outward. With this abatement of her "schizophrenic inertia," her omnipotent strivings, paranoid thinking, murderous rage toward oedipal rivals emerged in relation to the current social context with much heat. Therapeutic engagement was achieved. The timing of the therapist's transference confrontations was determined by observations made at many levels outside of the interview situation. Without these observations his awareness of transference developments would clearly have required an improbable sequence of highly intuitive guesses.

The usefulness of this expanded observational field is further highlighted by the fact that it facilitated an understanding of Gwen's regression during the tenth month and of her apparent improvement, so lacking in substance, during the sixteenth hospital month.

Insofar as the therapeutic community constitutes a highly cathected field for the elaboration, experiencing, and study of transferential behavior, an aspect of its therapeutic modus operandi is comprehensible in the psychodynamic frame of reference.

The many counterparts in our own clinical experience of the case presented here suggest the need for a reappraisal of the traditional belief that formulation and cure are bound by the sacrosanct confines of the one-to-one psychotherapeutic relationship.

SUMMARY

This paper describes a residential treatment approach that planfully employs the therapeutic community as an observational field upon which multiple transferences crystallize out. These transferences are studied and interpreted to the patient in an ongoing fashion in individual psychotherapeutic interviews. Using a variety of bound social contexts as vantage points, observations of the patient's transferentially determined behavior are systematically channeled to the therapist for synthesis with historical data and patient activity in the one-to-one psychotherapeutic relationship. The direct impact upon the patient of the affect arousal triggered by the social response to his transferential behavior serves to promote psychotherapeutic engagement and to catalyze the therapeutic process. This is viewed as an aspect of the therapeutic community's modus operandi which can be readily conceptualized in the psychodynamic frame of reference. Illustrative case material is presented in some detail.

REFERENCES

1. Schwartz, M., and Schwartz, C. G.: Considerations in Determining a Model for the Mental Hospital. *Am. J. Psychiat.,* 116: 435, 1959.
2. Grinker, R. R. A Transactional Model for Psychotherapy. *Arch. of Gen. Psychiat.,* 1: 132, 1959.
3. Hamburg, D.: Therapeutic Aspects of Communication and Administrative Policy in the Psychiatric Section of a General Hospital. In *Patient and the Mental Hospital,* Greenblatt, M., Levinson, D., and Williams, R., Eds. Free Press of Glencoe, Ill., 1957.
4. Jones, M.: The Treatment of Personality Disorders in a Therapeutic Community. *Psychiatry,* 20: 211, 1957.
5. Gough, H. G.: A Sociological Theory of Psychopathy. *Am. J. Sociol.* 53: 359, 1949.
6. Wilmer, Harry A.: Toward a Definition of the Therapeutic Community. *Am. J. Psychiat.,* 114: 9, 1958.
7. Scher, Jordan M.: The Structured Ward: Research Method and Hypothesis in a Total Treatment Setting for Schizophrenia. *Am. J. Orthopsychiat.,* 28: 2, 1958.
8. Candill, W., Redlich, F., Gilmore, H. and Brody E.: Social Structure and Interaction Process on a Psychiatric Ward. *Am. J. Orthopsychiat.,* 22: 314, 1952.
9. Gralnick, A. and D'Elia, F.: Role of the Patient in the Therapeutic Community. *Am. J. Psychother.,* 15: 63, 1961.
10. Cohen, R. A.: The Hospital as a Therapeutic Instrument. *Psychiatry,* 21: 29, 1958.
11. Denber, H. *Research Conf. on Therapeutic Community.* C. C Thomas, Springfield, Ill., 1959.
12. Redl, F.: Child Study in a New Setting. *Children,* 1: 15, 1954.
13. Saslow, G. and Meterrazo, J.: A Psychiatric Service in a General Hospital: A Setting for Social Learning. *Ment. Hosp.,* 13: 217, 1962.
14. Rabiner, E. L., Molinski, H. and Gralnick, A.: Conjoint Family Therapy in the Inpatient Setting. *Am. J. Psychother.,* 16: 618, 1962.

9

The Role of the Relative in a Psychotherapeutic Program: Anxiety Problems and Defensive Reactions Encountered

PAUL LEFEBVRE, M.D.
JUNIUS ATKINS, M.D.
JEROME DUCKMAN, M.D.
ALEXANDER GRALNICK, M.D.

IT IS EVIDENT from a study of the literature that the problem of dealing with the relatives of psychiatric patients has been recognized, but there remains a relative lack of organized information on this subject. Perhaps this is due to a generalized but often covert feeling among practitioners of psychotherapy that relatives constitute a hindrance to the effective treatment of mentally ill patients. As pointed out by Stanton and Schwartz,[5] such attitudes with regard to relatives often occur unconsciously in the therapist. On the other hand, many psychiatrists frankly state that dealing with relatives in any manner is detrimental to the effective management of the patient. Another source of obscurity about this subject lies in the fact that often what a therapist

This paper was read on May 14th, 1957, at the Annual Meeting of the American Psychiatric Association held in Chicago from May 13th, to 17th, 1957. Reprinted from *Canadian Psychiatric Association Journal,* Vol. III, No. 3, July, 1958, pp. 110-118.

does with regard to relatives is done on an intuitive basis, a situation which lends itself poorly to a clear formulation of what is being done.

At any rate, we have a growing awareness that there are advantages, but also problems to be encountered, in dealing with the relatives of mentally ill patients. Evidence of this trend is the current procedure of many child-guidance clinics of dealing therapeutically with both the child and one or both parents simultaneously. In the field of private practice with adult patients, psychotherapy of marriage partners has formed the object of a number of contributions.[4] Some workers[3] have reported on the positive merits of group therapy with the parents of schizophrenic patients.

The time has passed when responsibility for mental illness must be shouldered exclusively by the patient or his "constitution." Also, in the process of being discarded is the notion that the family alone, or the parents alone, are to blame for the occurrence of mental illness in the patient. In accord with the concept elaborated by Ackerman[1] we feel that the more realistic and current trend recognizes mental illness as a totalized process. This stresses the need to treat the patient and the family as a totalized unit. Succintly expressed, this represents an objective attiude that the patient and his family are a sick family and not merely a sick person who has a family. The family members, in this respect, are not seen as mere bystanders in the patient's illness. This constitutes the rationale for a therapeutic approach which seeks the family's useful participation and collaboration. Of this more will be said subsequently.

Our observations were made within the situational framework of High Point Hospital, a private, 45-bed psychiatric hospital. Almost all patients are admitted here on a voluntary basis. The senior staff consists of psychoanalytically trained psychiatrists. The treatment emphasis is on intensive psychoanalytically oriented psychotherapy with the shock and drug therapies used adjunctively. All varieties of psychiatric disorders are represented in the patient population, although the majority of the patients are schizophrenics, many of them borderline cases. There is no separate social service department and all dealings with relatives are carried on by the therapists themselves. Most of the patients belong to an upper-middle class level of urban society, many with an educational background of college level. Since High Point Hospital counts among its patients a majority of schizophrenics, for whom long-term, intensive psychotherapy is often the treatment of choice, we believe that an adequate period of hospitalization is highly desirable for the patient's welfare. Inasmuch as many of the problems encountered with relatives concern the maintenance of hospitalization, the therapist, who, through his contacts with the relatives, has contributed to such maintenance, has by the same token enhanced the patient's chances for recovery.

If personal dealings with relatives are to have their maximum value, the objective has to be more comprehensive than merely utilizing them as sources of historical and collateral information about the patient. However, this objective remains entirely valid and fruitful. Particularly with schizophrenic patients is this true, because of the frequent distortions they make both in their thinking and reporting. Through the acquisition and scrutiny of collateral information, one can discern not only gross but even subtle manifestations of paranoid thinking, grandiosity and other psychopathological features. It is of course true that in many instances facts or situations as reported by relatives contain a variable amount of distortion, just as one observes in therapeutic transactions with patients. This very fact, however, permits one to obtain revealing glimpses of the family dynamics in action. Furthermore, with the opportunity of repeated contacts with the family, the therapist is enabled, in spite of the distortions in the data offered by the patient and the relatives, to make accurate, personal formulations as to what, in any given situation, actually occurred. We are inclined to stress the importance for the therapist of repeated contacts with the relatives as a simple means of obtaining historical data along with significant discrepancies therein. Also, this permits fruitful observations concerning the dynamics of the family as a whole, and the particular patterns of interaction of the patient himself within the family unit.

There are other valid objectives which a therapist has in dealing with relatives. By and large, most families as a unit are fundamentally interested in behaving in the patient's best interests. This remains true in spite of the fact that what the relative believes to be best for the patient may not coincide with the patient's actual needs. One also knows of course that a relative can constitute, wittingly or unwittingly, an influence upon the patient that is quite destructive. However, since relatives generally are desirous of participating in some way in the total treatment situation of the patient, the therapist naturally seeks to insure that their participation will be beneficial rather than detrimental to the patient's treatment. This requires the therapist to have sufficient contact with the relatives so that he may evaluate which is most constructively inclined, and recognize and control destructive tendencies in others.

Contacts with relatives are also of value in alleviating their countless anxieties through the giving of proper information and the correction of misconceptions. More will be said of this subsequently.

In spite of the importance we have placed on therapist-family contacts, we tend to temper enthusiasm with a realization that only limited goals may be achieved in dealing with relatives. We avoid extravagant expectations of lasting attitudinal or behavioral changes in the relatives. It is occasionally possible, however, to make therapeutic use of this very fact, as we will attempt to illustrate with a later case in point.

Relatives, generally speaking, when faced with the prospect of mental illness in the family, manifest anxiety, and defensiveness as a response to this very anxiety. These responses of relatives constitute primary problems which have to be dealt with in working with them. Naturally a working understanding of the sources of the anxiety in particular relatives is helpful.

ANXIETY

We will not attempt to explore all the known causes of the anxieties of relatives, but rather to mention some of the more obvious ones, and elaborate on some others which in our experience have appeared particularly significant or troublesome.

Shame with regard to mental illness, a sense of personal or family stigma, are still prevalent, in spite of all the efforts to increase public understanding and tolerance. This sense of shame is sometimes openly stated, more often it is merely implied. Yet it rarely fails to provoke anxiety in relatives, and various defensive operations which are sometimes quite detrimental to the patient's welfare. This occurs for example when shame impels the relative to minimize if not to deny the very existence let alone the gravity of the mental illness in the patient.

Relatives will often develop anxiety because of guilt feelings concerning their at least dimly felt participation in the causation of the patient's illness.

Even today, one encounters anxiety in relatives in connection with fearsome expectations that mental illness is hereditary and that it will be transmitted to the patient's offspring. Yet another observable cause of anxiety in relatives is the feeling that mental illness is incurable, and that little hope can be held for the patient's eventual improvement or recovery. In the case of a previously untreated patient, anxiety in relatives may result from their feeling negligent in not recognizing the existence, the nature or the gravity of the patient's illness.

Relatives often show anxious perplexity in the face of the patient's illness and quite openly confess a more or less complete lack of understanding of "what it is all about." This is a reaction which all too frequently provokes in the therapist an unfortunate tendency to develop an ambivalent, often critical attitude toward the relative.[5] This often is related to the therapist's covert tendency to identify with the patient. The nature of such responses to relatives on the part of the therapist is not difficult to unmask. This is more in the nature of true transference since the therapist is unwittingly reacting to the patient's relatives as very often he might to his own. This is in contrast to the usual countertransference response in which the therapist irrationally and without awareness responds to an irrational stimulus provided by the patient himself. The therapist who deals directly with relatives must always be mindful of the fact that psychological illness is after all an extremely complex and only partially understood process. The average relative cannot then be expected to show any great amount of objective understanding of the patient's illness. This is true above and beyond the fact that relatives lack true understanding because of their emotional involvement with the patient.

A phenomenon which is also observable as a source of anxiety in relatives when a patient is admitted to a psychiatric hospital is the dawning awareness that he or she is threatened with having to adjust to or live with a psychotic person. This can be observed to create a diffuse anxiety, which at times is quite overwhelming to the relative. We recollect the uncanny dread momentarily experienced by a husband who had come to recognize the gravity of his wife's illness. He stated: "My God, what did I marry . . ."

Relatives are made anxious by the financial shift that results when the family breadwinner is incapacitated by mental illness, and another family member is faced with the responsibility of providing for the family in whole or in part. The lowering of the total family income due to the cost of hospitalization and the disappearance of savings intended for schooling or old age are all sources of anxiety.

Certainly the major and most complex factor related to the anxiety of relatives is the withdrawal through hospitalization of the ill person and whatever emotional needs he supplies to the other family members. When this occurs, one needs to be alertly observant of the manner in which the patient and one relative or more struggle to maintain a form of mutual interpersonal balance, a certain implicit homeostatic arrangement one with the other. Under close scrutiny this invariably is seen to have existed for a long time. It has been spoken of, especially with regard to schizophrenics, as a symbiotic process between the patient and the relative. Lewis Hill[2] has made an interesting contribution to the understanding of this problem in his remarks about the "schizophrenogenic mother."

Hospitalization, because of the threat it produces to this morbid symbiotic balance between patient and relative, often constitutes in itself a source of considerable anxiety in relatives.

The following represents a dramatic illustration of the interpersonal balance described, although in this example the reactive change in the relative occurred in the form of an unusual improvement in physical functioning.

Case 1: B.S., a 42 year old married physician, was hospitalized in an acute state of pan-anxiety of schizophrenic proportions. The patient's pre-morbid personality was characterized by marked schizoid features and a great deal of sustained dependency towards his parents, especially his mother. The patient's mother had exercised a high degree of influence over the patient through the medium of chronic complaint, usually of a somatic nature. Three years before, the patient's mother began to complain bitterly of symptoms referrable to rheumatoid arthritis. The patient became quite concerned, made arrangements to have his parents move from a distant section of the city into an apartment in the same building in which the patient practiced. Thereafter, he treated his mother assiduously, in spite of which she led the life of a partial invalid. The patient persisted in treating his mother, although she presented only symptoms of the illness, without physical or radiographic evidence of arthritis. This occurred in spite of the fact that the patient was a well-qualified internist and a rather meticulous diagnostician. When the patient became mentally ill, his mother began to show dramatic freedom from arthritic complaint and blossomed physically. The observation of this phenomenon increased the therapist's understanding by crystallizing the warped nature of the patient's relationship with his mother, and permitted further therapeutic exploration of it. This same patient would characteristically confide most of his own family's even commonplace difficulties to his parents, in spite of his awareness that they would worry themselves to excess and telephone the patient several times a day for reassurance that all was well. In spite of his awareness of the irrational character of his morbid dependence, the patient persisted in this practice, often incurring the critical disapproval of his wife. This compulsive tendency to confide in his parents evidently corresponded to a morbid need in this patient. Conversely his mother's ability to obtain the patient's constant medical attention to her varied physical complaints constituted a veritable, largely unconscious "devil's bargain," whereby there was silent agreement that each would tolerate the irrationality of the other in order to gratify their symbiotic needs. As this situation grew clearer, it became possible to explore the morbid aspects of this relationship further.

DEFENSIVENESS

Most of the problems encountered in dealing with relatives stem from the defensiveness they show with respect to their fears and anxieties about the hospitalized family member. The defensiveness of relatives manifests itself in a variety of more or less troublesome reactions. We would like to single out a few which have commanded our special attention.

One type of relative tends to engage in rather overt obstructionism with regard to the treatment program of the patient. The following case will illustrate this point.

Case 2.: Mrs. F. R., a 32-year old married female, was admitted with a history of having suffered recurring bouts of depression, anxiety, severe phobic reactions and vague feelings of unreality over a period of one year. Although in psychiatric treatment for many months prior to admission, this patient over the objections of her husband and her therapist took the initiative of admitting herself to High Point Hospital, feeling that she could no longer "cope with the situation." In reality Mrs. R. had sensed the dreadful imminence of overpowering panic and had been able to mobilize enough motivation to seek hospitalization. With time a diagnosis of schizophrenia was made. The patient's husband, from the onset, was unable to grasp the gravity of his wife's condition. Contrary to advice he exerted great pressure to take his wife off the grounds for more or less prolonged absences from the hospital. When this occurred, the patient invariably experienced an aggravation of her symptomatology, which however did not deter Mr. R. from maintaining his pressure. His own great anxiety made him attempt to prove that she was "not so sick" by having her do what we knew she was not ready for. Attempts to work with Mr. R. on this problem revealed only that his anxiety would not permit him to modify his destructive behavior, and that too emphatic disagreement on our part would provoke him into bringing about the premature discharge of the patient. It was therefore elected to tolerate some of his ill-advised demands whenever we felt no lasting harm to the patient would ensue. These enforced outings continued to be followed by periods of severe anxiety. Finally Mr. R. recognized much more than he had that his demands and behavior were detrimental to the patient. Concurrently, this situation was dealt with in therapy and it became apparent to Mrs. R. that the ill-advised outings increased her distress. In time the patient became able to assume a more self-protective and asserting role with her husband. With such a method of handling the situation, the patient remained in treatment sufficiently long so that she could leave considerably improved, although some minor difficulties with Mrs. R. persisted throughout.

It might be added, incidentally, that Mr. R. on his first contact with the patient's therapist, offered the latter a "gift." It has been our experience that a relative who does so at the onset of treatment can usually be expected to bargain for some "favor" from the therapist.

The following case illustrates how obstructionism on the part of a relative can be manifested in a less direct yet no less destructive fashion. In this instance, the relative, while quite aware of the nature of her behavior, nevertheless intruded herself and her opinions into the therapeutic situation in a manner detrimental to the patient's welfare.

Case 3: B. R., a 22-year old unmarried female, was classified prior to her admission to High Point Hospital, as a dependent-aggressive personality. A previous hospitalization, following a suicidal attempt, lasted but one week, because of the mother's irresponsible intervention. Later, ten months of psychotherapy as an out-patient proved unproductive and in the face of increasing depression the patient received a total of 40 electro-convulsive treatments on an ambulatory basis. The patient's former therapist complained of the persistent sabotage of his therapeutic efforts by the patient's mother, and when the patient was admitted to High Point we could soon agree with him.

From the outset the mother was reluctant to give up the idea that she could do more for her daughter than any psychiatrist. In spite of our advice to the contrary, she persisted in her exhortations that the patient "buck up and get better." The mother, in this respect, challenged the patient, argued with her, and embarrassed her on visiting days by disparaging her efforts at improvement. Whenever the therapist was able to help the patient make plainly observable gains, the patient's mother found some relatively minor point to complain about, such as: "But, Doctor, you are doing nothing about my daughter's excessive weight . . ." On occasion she would express satisfaction with the patient's progress in the therapist's presence, only to later disparage him when alone with the patient. It became clear that this parent felt her symbiotic relationship with the patient threatened by any move towards improvement on the part of the patient.

Rather typically, the patient's father had been quite inconspicuous and unassuming. He was gradually activated in this situation. The therapist's tactic proved auspicious inasmuch as the father was found capable, with encouragement and support, of counteracting the unwholesome maternal influence. Despite the initial unwarranted plaint that hospitalization was too expensive to be borne, the parents, because of the more active role assumed by the father, soon were in agreement with a long-term treatment. The patient then concurred, particularly as the mother's unwise pressure abated. The consideration of expense was placed in proper perspective. The irrational aspects of the behavior of both mother and patient were brought into therapeutic focus. Released from undue pressure the patient recognized her faulty patterns and explored the ambivalent attitudes toward her mother which had created her dependent-aggressive traits. The mother became increasingly tolerant of the therapist's efforts, although hardly a paragon of cooperation. The father's role grew increasingly important. His mobilization played no small part in achieving a smoother relationship with the mother in a manner which proved quite encouraging to the patient. We have found it a valuable practice in our experience, when one parent is a real problem to involve the other parent more actively in the treatment program, even if he originally seemed a relatively passive and inadequate person.

The following case, too, is an example of "defensive obstructionism." However, in this instance the response was provoked by any evidence of progress on the part of the patient in the face of the prognosis originally determined to be very poor.

Case 4: Mrs. B. K., was a 41-year old hebephrenic whose husband, a physician, had developed an over-pessimistic attitude at the onset of her illness, finally concluding that she would have to be committed to a state hospital. His attitude was not modified by the fact that her identical twin had overcome a paranoid schizophrenic episode. He had already removed her prematurely from several hospitals, and from the care of a number of psychiatrists until her siblings actively intervened in the immediate period before her admission to High Point, and insisted that she finally be hospitalized for a fair period of time. Their intervention was encouraged by the referring psychiatrist who had continued to treat her despite her husband's protests. The patient's hebephrenic symptoms had returned in force, and her husband would have preferred she be committed to a state hospital.

When Mrs. B. K. was admitted to High Point in June, 1955, her husband seemed willing to cooperate despite his attitude of hopelessness and his wish for her commitment to a state institution. At the third month, when she definitely was showing progress, her husband began threatening to take her out of the hospital because of the financial burden. The patient's family revealed at this time that actually he was not involved since they had been providing the funds for her care. His next gesture was to observe and use any symptoms still present in the patient to argue for discontinuation of treatment on the basis of futility. However, at this time, he was not quite willing to take full responsibility for her. Subsequently he sought cooperation by seeking sympathy for himself. In order to prevent his interference a separation agreement was proposed and her family agreed to assume full responsibility. With this, he withdrew, and the patient began to improve rapidly. She established reasonable goals, found a job and reestablished her previous relationship with the referring psychiatrist. The patient was then discharged considerably improved in March, 1956.

We have observed that in attempting to enlist the constructive participation of relatives in a therapeutic program, realism compels that goals remain relative and modest. With an awareness of the complexly symbiotic needs of both relative and patient, it is unrealistic to expect too durable modifications of attitude and attendant behavior in the relative. This is so in spite of the occurrence of some favorable changes in the latter at the onset of hospitalization or the onset of illness. To be sure, one may observe a relative, who had for many years shown a significantly destructive lack of empathy for the patient, react with consideration and concern, but by and large the permanency of such changes is best kept in thoughtful doubt.

The following case is an illustration of this fact, and the manner in which it came to be used to therapeutic advantage.

Case 5: Mrs. G. B., a 30-year old schizophrenic, was a patient in long-term psychotherapy at High Point. She had been progressing satisfactorily and appeared encouraged when her husband began to show modification of certain attitudes and behavior which had previously constituted for her a source of chronic dissatisfaction. After a time, however, the patient's husband gradually began to revert to type. The patient herself was in complete disagreement with his sudden decision that she leave the hospital, and she accordingly became increasingly depressed. She was helped to see that her husband's previous and reassuring change was proving illusory, and that if her life situation was to improve in any meaningful sense, the onus of change would ultimately rest upon her. This was a difficult fact for the patient to grasp and accept but eventually Mrs. B. was able to take a more direct approach to her husband and successfully insist that her position was correct. This proved to be a novel response for this patient, and one which represented a healthy step.

Hostile interaction between one member of the marital unit and a member or more of the patient's peripheral family (siblings or parents) may be a source of anxiety that proves troublesome to the therapeutic process.

Case 6: Such a case was that of Mrs. D. K., a twice-married 35-year old dentist's wife, who was admitted in December, 1955, with an acute paranoid schizophrenia. At this time her brothers and sisters were violently denunciatory of her husband, blaming him for her illness. In accord with them was a neuro-psychiatrist, Mrs. D. K.'s friend, who was certain the patient would never get well if the marriage were not terminated immediately. The husband gave every indication that he felt a certain amount of hostility toward the patient. Solution of this problem was impossible until the patient had recovered sufficiently to discuss her relationships with both her husband and her family. Then she revealed how her family's attitude had developed previous to her breakdown. She, being unable to express hostile feelings toward her husband, had communicated them by certain nonverbal methods. These communications stimulated her family to express her hostile feelings toward her husband for her (and vice versa) while she sat back, listened and felt innocently relieved. But she had fanned her family's hostility to such a pitch that she had become fearful of what might happen to her marriage. They had begun to demand that she divorce her husband. He was drinking more and staying out longer in response to their attitude. Then the patient became ill. There was no doubt that this marriage was superior to the patient's previous one. Noteworthy, too, is the fact that criticism of the marriage was limited to two areas—the husband's heavy drinking and irregular periods of absenteeism from home in the evenings.

When the patient responded poorly in the first two months at High Point, her family's anxiety, and resentment of her husband increased. At this point her brothers forced her husband by threats of physical violence to admit all the blame. This relieved their anxiety but was otherwise of no help.

With an understanding of the patient's ability to provoke hostility between the patient's husband and peripheral family, it was possible to eliminate this as a source of intra-family anxiety (for the husband had actually begun to act hostilely toward her because of her family's treatment of him.) As the patient now reassured her family, their feeling of futility about the situation disappeared together with the logical anxiety. Their attitude toward her husband improved, as did his toward the patient. Further improvement continued, and the patient was discharged in May, 1956.

In order to avoid the impression that relatives invariably respond to their anxieties in a manner detrimental to the patient, we append the following case to illustrate how one may unwittingly ignore the judgment of a level-headed, informed relative.

Case 7: M. L., was a 49-year old divorced female who had for many years prior to admission suffered severe compulsive symptoms and phobic reactions. From the moment she entered the hospital this patient was extremely critical of everything and everyone about her. Her manner was irrationally bitter. The patient's brother had been able to remain quite objective about her illness, and was eager to have her receive prolonged treatment. The patient soon became rather ingratiating with her therapist, indicating that if it were not for him her stay at the hospital would be unbearable. She gradually showed signs of "improvement," seemed to engage in therapy, and change her critical attitude. She stated that she now would not think of leaving the hospital until her therapist agreed she was well enough. At a later date the patient applied for permission to spend a week-end at home because of an important holiday. The brother was consulted and expressed some anxiety about the end result of the projected visit. The therapist, failing to recognize this as well-founded anxiety, reassured the brother that the patient was gratified at her progress and would not refuse to return. She was allowed to go with the inevitable result that once there she decided to remain at home. Hind-sight, of course, is better than fore-sight, but had the therapist recognized this relative's anxiety for what it really was he would have properly re-evaluated the patient's "progress" as a highly manipulative maneuver. The visit would have been disallowed, and interruption of therapy prevented.

It is therefore important to identify that relative in a family who seems the most objective and be alert to the validity of his anxiety and the help it offers the psychotherapeutic program.

SUMMARY AND CONCLUSIONS

This paper describes a number of observations made by the medical staff of this hospital in its dealings with the relatives of our patients subjected to an intensive psychotherapeutic program.

Our frame of reference has been the recognition of mental illness as a totalized process, involving the family as a psycho-social unit. Hospitalization of one family member is observed to provoke in relatives a number of reactions which can be summarized as anxiety and defensive operations against such anxiety. The latter characteristically create the various problems a therapist encounters and must solve in order to insure that the relatives' participation in the treatment program will prove beneficial rather than detrimental to the patient.

The importance, particularly with psychotic patients, of having repeated therapist-relative contacts has been stressed. We have found them beneficial to the patient's effective treatment.

We believe that only limited goals may be sought in

working with relatives since lasting attitudinal and behavioral changes are not common, although certain limited modifications along these lines may be achieved.

The paper, further, reviews some of the known sources of anxiety in the relatives of hospitalized psychiatric patients.

A number of troublesome defensive operations against anxiety have been illustrated with case material.

While we appreciate that this report constitutes a very modest contribution to an understanding of the relatives of psychiatric patients, we do hope that it will stimulate further investigation of this important topic.

BIBLIOGRAPHY

1. Ackerman, N.: "Interpersonal Disturbances in the Family," Psychiatry (1954) 17: 359-368.
2. Hill, L.: "Psychotherapeutic Intervention in Schizophrenia," Univ. of Chicago Press, Chicago, 1955, pp. 100-132.
3. Kahn, S. and Prestwood, A. R.: "Group Psychotherapy of Parents as an Adjunct to the Treatment of Schizophrenic Patients," Psychiatry (1954) 17: 177-186.
4. Martin, P. and Bird, H. W.: "An Approach to the Psychotherapy of Marriage Partners." Psychiatry (1953) 16: 123-128.
5. Stanton, A. H. and Schwartz, M. S.: "The Mental Hospital," Basic Books, Inc., New York, 1954, pp. 98-99-100.

10

Family Psychotherapy: General and Specific Considerations

ALEXANDER GRALNICK, M.D.

Family psychotherapy is increasingly accepted as a form of treatment. This article reviews some of its history, rationale and theoretical bases. A definition of family psychotherapy is offered and the suggestion made that at this early time we be as objective as possible about the subject. Hospital experience which led to the practice of family psychotherapy with the inpatient is described, as well as its aims. The role of the family therapist, techniques of treatment, results and general propositions are discussed.

FAMILY PSYCHOTHERAPY, simply put, is the nonorganic psychiatric treatment of the sick family. In this sentence the simplicity of the subject begins and ends, for further reflection brings to mind a host of matters. These would include such things as a more comprehensive definition, the anlages of the subject as well as its history, its rationale, its value, techniques of its application, and the exploration of one's experience with it.

The psychiatrist who undertakes the treatment of a patient has wittingly, or unwittingly, committed himself to

---

Presented at a professional meeting held by the Haven Sanitarium in Detroit, Michigan, December 3, 1960. Reprinted from *The American Journal of Orthopsychiatry,* Vol. XXXII, No. 3, April, 1962, pp. 515-526.

affecting the lives of a family. This is true whether he sees members of the family other than the patient or not, for they think of and react to him in their everyday living with the patient. The therapist may be alternately a respected, loved or hated figure, depending on the manner in which the behavior of the treated member affects the others. In some respects the therapist becomes an adopted or incorporated member of the group. This is a role that can neither be discounted nor evaded by denial of its existence. Almost by its own weight such a situation makes the acceptance and practice of family psychotherapy quite logical.

It is a fact, however, that family psychotherapy—at least, in any conscious and defined manner—did not come upon the scene concurrently with individual psychotherapy, no matter how logic would have indicated that this should have been the case. As a matter of fact, particularly with the introduction of psychoanalytic principles, the idea of seeing members of a patient's family, let alone treating them, was looked upon as strange, if not heretical, until rather recent years.

It is probably fair to say that as soon as psychoanalysts began to deviate from strictly orthodox technique the seeds were planted for present-day analytic psychotherapy of the family. When the therapist injected himself, as a person, into the therapeutic relationship, the groundwork was laid for broadening his interest in the patient to eventually include his family. The patient, then, was no longer an isolate, only related to his family biologically and instinctually, but interactionally, as part of a social unit with its own dynamics. The growth of group psychotherapy and its apparent value was another forerunner of family psychotherapy. This form of treatment made evident the fact that a group of people has dynamics and pathodynamics similar to those which are present in a family. If therapy could affect its members positively, it took little further imagination to conceive of therapy of the family itself. I think the concept of milieu therapy and the therapeutic community in the treatment of inpatients probably also made up part of the groundwork for the practice of family psychotherapy.

One historical fact might be mentioned at this point which has some bearing on the growing acceptance of family psychotherapy. Psychoanalysis has outgrown its infancy. The wave of enthusiasm which marked its initial years has passed its crest. Many of its pioneers have gone from the scene, taking with them the zeal which originally suffused the psychoanalytic movement. It had been natural for them to look to this new knowledge to conquer the frustrating illnesses with which they had been grappling. This is in the nature of things in psychiatry. Added years of experience, however, have indicated the rather narrow limits of effectiveness of strict psychoanalytic procedure, and have revealed a distressing recurrence of illness in treated patients. Under such conditions it was natural for the idea of family psychotherapy—as an innovation—to have appeal even for the most avid psychoanalyst, particularly since many of the basic tenets of psychoanalysis could be preserved.

Although it may be said that when the first psychiatrist took a history from a family member of his patient, family psychotherapy was initiated, it is more exact, from the evidence, to see it as having begun in more recent years. As sociologists, anthropologists, and other social scientists contributed to the interdisciplinary approach, the main focus of interest moved to the family itself. The earliest workers who may be said to have truly engaged in family therapy were those who began to work with married couples. Among the first was the well-known analyst, Clarence Oberndorf,[1] who, in 1934, reported on his experience in treating a marital pair. In the 1940's, Mittelman[2,3] began to report on his work with series of couples, indicating that he saw them simultaneously or separately, depending on conditions. He indicated that it was important for the therapist to be impartial and of good will, and to demonstrate that he wished to dispel misunderstanding between the two. Otherwise, he cautioned the therapist hardy enough to engage in such work not to be neutral, to avoid being too free with his opinion, and to instruct the mates neither to discuss their analyses nor to quote the analyst. We may imagine how revolutionary this type of practice was at that time, and how difficult it was for those who attempted it in the face of contrary tradition and principle.

In the early 1950's, Mittelman[4] began to report on the simultaneous treatment of both parents and their children. He said such treatment was advantageous, and sometimes indispensable for the best therapeutic results. Along about this time child psychiatrists were reporting efforts to treat the whole family in their attempt to solve the child's problems.

In 1953, Martin and Bird[5] described the close cooperation of therapists treating respective mates of a marriage. In addition to seeing their countertransference reactions more easily they saw such advantages as the following: 1) a saving of time, 2) a better chance to evaluate their therapy, 3) a better opportunity to time and coordinate interpretaions and progress, and to perceive warning signs of impending trouble. Reporting on the treatment of eight couples in 1956, Thomas[6] stated that the therapist has to assume an attitude of ignorance of the second mate when seeing the first. This certainly would seem to be a tall order. He points out, further, that in this type of treatment situation, the transference relationship becomes secondary and the emphasis shifts from the therapeutic to the marriage relationship.

In recent years the more serious work in family psychotherapy has been done by Ackerman, Bowen, Grotjahn and Jackson. Time will not permit any detailed account of their respective work, except to say that they are engaged with the actual treatment of the family as a unit, including children, rather than merely the couple.

It would seem that certain ideas would have to be taken for granted if one would hope to undertake family psychotherapy in comfort. First, that the individual is not an isolate but an effective member of a group who acts and interacts with the others. Second, that family interrelationships are highly complex, and that there are multiple orders of interaction within the family. Third, that patient-family-member relationships are of equal importance as patient-therapist ones. Fourth, that the study of and insight into the nature of these relationships can be therapeutic without awareness of one's libidinal drives, and without the production of a transference neurosis. Fifth, that the study of current experience within the family group is as important as the study of early life experiences and the "origins" of pathology, not only for the improvement of the individual, but also for the general well-being of the group. Sixth, that the family group has its own psychopathology apart from and different from the individual's. It is to this pathology that we may address ourselves, and once having improved it, affect the individual's psychopathology secondarily, without having necessarily assaulted it primarily and directly. This is accomplished by the therapist's own action in the group, whereas in individual therapy the therapist's action is directly on the patient's pathology. When the latter is resolved, the patient may effect changes in the family's psychopathology by his own actions. Seventh, that the patient has responsibilities to the group as such, and to its respective members individually, and that in turn the group, as a unit, has responsibility to the individual member, as such. This last idea—and belief—is more apparent to the family therapist than to the individual therapist, and the patient's pathology, studied right within the group, is made more apparent more readily.

Apart from seeming to have a degree of necessity, family psychotherapy has a certain rationale. We in psychiatry—at least those of us who are psychoanalytically oriented—start with the assumption that the family is a small social unit which originates the emotional life of its members, and that the quality of this emotional life stems from the nature of the human interrelationships which exist therein. Though some of us may believe, additionally, that behavior may have biological determinants, we are more convinced that it, as well as emotions, is determined by the structure and dynamics of the family itself. As Ackerman[7] says, the family is a social system and we "must think of the person not in isolation, but rather as part of this social system." When it is put this way, one cannot help but wonder why we did not start with the actual treatment of the family promptly upon the introduction of psychoanalyic theory and practice. I suppose the reasons are multiple. Freud himself apparently could not handle family members of patients, and advised that they be kept as far from the therapeutic scene as possible. One can only speculate to what extent his difficulties flowed from theoretical formulations, and to what degree from countertransference problems. We do know, however, the great influence that countertransference may have on theoretical constructions. At any rate, the very system of thinking that found the origins of pathology in family relationships (biologically determined, it is true, rather than socially) proscribed the active treatment of the family unit as such. Perhaps in the earlier years the treatment of a single individual was complicated and difficult enough. Perhaps, as already indicated, the breadth of our experience and vision had to await expansion. Certainly, in the current era, more of us seem to accept the proposition increasingly, and feel up to the task of treating the family.

If the origins of mental illness reside within the family, it would seem that the resolution of psychopathology lies there too. After all, the individual does not carry his illness in some encapsulated form, but demonstrates it in action with people, probably most acutely with members of his family. What better place then to make the most accurate observation of pathology and to bring therapeutic influence to bear most decisively? What better place to add the presence and personality of the skilled, learned and rational therapist? It would seem like the addition of some ingredient to the brew which changes its quality and consistency.

The aims of individual and family psychotherapy are alike, namely the alteration of human behavior through the intervention of another human being. Individual psychotherapy needs no definition here. We can, however, attempt to define family psychotherapy. I say "attempt" because as yet there is no clearly defined understanding of exactly what it is, who is included in the process, how we go about practicing it, precisely what we are looking for in the way of pathology, or specifically what our goal, the healthy family, is. Ackerman is inclined to regard family therapy as such only if it includes the entire family unit, that is, at least the parents and children, in joint sessions with one and the same therapist. His definition permits the therapist additionally to see individual members of the family. I did hear him say recently that seeing a marital pair is not family therapy, and that the therapy of different members of a family by separate therapists is not such therapy either. The latter type of treatment situation is usually referred to as collaborative therapy when the therapists confer with each other about their respective patients. Jackson[8] refers to seeing the patient and parents, and possibly siblings too, at one and the same time, as conjoint therapy, and limits the term "family therapy" to "family oriented collaborative psychotherapy, where family members are seen in individual psychotherapy." Martin and Bird[5] describe the collaborative technique of two therapists who treat respective marital partners as the "stereoscopic" technique. Thus, we have stereoscopic family therapy.

It would seem that in the present stage of our knowledge we cannot afford to be too dogmatic in our definition of family therapy. For the moment it would seem sufficient if we more universally agreed that this type of approach to the treatment of patients is valuable enough to adopt with little reservation. The stricter definition and techniques would then evolve out of the greater experience we have with it. Personally, I would favor describing as family therapy any psychotherapeutic approach to the primary patient which consciously included other members of his family, seen either separately or jointly with the primary patient. The definition would include a situation in which the same or more therapists were involved in the treatment of the family members, so long as there was collaboration by the therapists, and would hold whether the entire family were involved or not, although it would seem preferable if the entire family were involved conjointly, at least sometimes. Naturally, the definition could only hold if a therapeutic effect were sought for all of the members as individuals, as well as for the family as a social unit—not just for the primary patient.

I suppose that everyone who engages in the serious practice of family therapy, in any of its forms, has had a certain experiential background which leads to his accepting it. Ackerman's interest in the subject stems from psychoanalytic training and teaching, experience with family agencies, the practice of individual and group psychotherapy as an ego psychologist, and intimate contact with experts in related disciplines. Grotjahn[9] states that only when he saw the wives of student analysands, who tended to treat their analysis intellectually, would progress be made. This experience started him on family therapy. In a recent unpublished paper Jackson says that the analyst who engages in family therapy must be prepared to be influenced by the experience. The family therapist, he says, finds himself emphasizing the current scene rather than the past, the interactional rather than the intrapsychic, and soon sees himself taking an increasingly active role in therapy. I myself would guess that the therapist who engages in family therapy has already seen the value, and been an adherent of such practices in individual therapy, and it is this, among other things, that has led him to family therapy where, of course, experience makes them even more logical.

After this rather lengthy introduction, I shall present some of our experiences at High Point Hospital in the field of family psychotherapy. Having indicated that those who engage in it have a particular background and approach I would be less than fair if I neglected to report my own to you, even at the expense of appearing self-indulgent or self-laudatory. My first seven to eight years of work in psychiatry were spent in the more-or-less typical State Hospital, with an exposure to the type of experience with which you are all familiar. Like most others, I regarded the family primarily as a source of historical data. Though rather sympathetically inclined toward him, I recall unwillingness to spend more time with the family member than was necessary, other than to instruct and help him to understand the patient a bit. There were social workers to see the family member and I was busy. The idea that any opportunity resided here for family therapy was completely foreign to me, even though during the latter four years of my stay there I was engaged concurrently in my psychoanalytic training.

During the succeeding five years of private psychoanalytic practice, I was the typical therapist who treasured his intimate relation with his patients to the virtual exclusion of their relatives. True, my patients generally were the usual neurotic individuals whose problems were hardly so acute as to warrant calling in the relative. Or so it always appeared. However, now as I look back it seems to me that some of my patients, and their families, might very well have fared better had I done some joint work with them. At the time, the tradition of keeping the patient's secret and the fear of threatening the precious transference relationship were undoubtedly too much for me to overcome.

When I undertook to organize and direct High Point Hospital some ten years ago things did change, to say the very least. For the moment I will not speculate or expound on what might have moved me from the comforts of an office psychoanalytic practice into the nature of my current work. I like to believe, and remember, that sometimes I felt I was not doing quite enough for my patients or quite enough for a larger number of sicker people. I like to feel that my training, experience and personal inclination were having something of a logical development, and that I could make a contribution appropriate to it. Perhaps it was simply the nature of my personality, unrelated to anything else.

At any rate, the inpatient care of borderline and psychotic patients with intensive psychoanalytically oriented psychotherapy presented an entirely different set of circumstances, and a new perspective determined by experiences quite different from those enjoyed in office practice. In the first place, the patient is both sicker and more-or-less completely dependent upon the relative for emotional and economic support. The family member now feels in a much stronger position vis-à-vis the psychiatrist, as well as the patient. Since the situation is more desperate than when the patient was in ambulatory therapy, the relative can "demand" to see the therapist. Previously the parent was helpless when refused access to the therapist because the patient was self-sufficient; now the roles were reversed. In fact, the parent begins to hold the whip hand because he holds the purse strings, and can place the patient where he himself will get a more sympathetic ear. In his opinion the office psychiatrist had been short-sighted in not seeing him, the parent, and the proof of this is quite evident, for the patient has decompensated and required hospitalization. Under these circumstances the parent is not going to be denied his need again.

On his part, the hospital therapist dealing with a more acute problem, finds he needs the relative, at least for history, and certainly for more than that if he wishes to treat the patient intensively. Therefore, a train of reality factors forces the therapist and relative together, no matter how resentful and suspicious they may be of each other initially. If they both have the welfare of the patient as their main goal, however, and keep open minds—and hearts—family psychotherapy must be born. And so it is! And so it was with us! One might say it has a scientific logic, for a certain set of circumstances have developed upon which are brought to bear the experiences of specific human beings, namely the relative and therapist. They can do nothing else but engage together with the patient in achieving their common goal—the restoration of the patient's health.

One other factor was present in the Hospital's earliest stages of development which perhaps contributed to the growth of family therapy in our institution—and that was a very limited budget. As a consequence we could not employ a social worker. The end result was that there was no intermediary between therapist and relative. They had to meet frequently if anything basic was to be accomplished for the patient. As we made the observations yet to be recounted, what started as the result of economic circumstance became a matter of therapeutic policy—namely, that all communications between family and therapist be direct.

The psychiatrist who spends much time with relatives of patients is likely to develop a sympathetic attitude toward them, no matter what his previous approach may have been. He soon finds that many are as disturbed as the patients themselves, but that more are positively motivated toward the patient than not. What is very obvious is that most of them, despite the best of intentions, are quite uninformed about the most elementary problems of the patient, and consequently quite helpless. They have certainly had little previous assistance from anyone—particularly of a sympathetic nature. As a rule, the relative believes that he has been considered the bête noire by both the patient and psychiatrist. When the hospital therapist meets him with a show of concern for his own difficulties, and with evident belief in his good intention toward the patient, the relative will rather easily enter into a good working relationship with the therapist. I believe that the good individual therapist has sympathy for the patient he elects to treat. To the extent that the hospitalized patient's therapist has sympathy for the patient's family, to that extent can he encourage and enter into family therapy with them.

We at High Point have many avenues of contact and communication with the family either separately or together with the patient. Ordinarily some significant member of the family brings the patient to the Hospital for admission. At this very time the family will establish contact with the hospital therapists both separately and jointly with the patient. Face-to-face contact is supplemented by frequent telephonic and written communication. This type of communication is also supplemented by the "contact" a therapist has through the verbal description patients give of the relative, and which administrative staff, in contact with the relative, will give of him. All of this, plus numerous interviews, tends to establish a rather thorough contact between the therapist and relative.

I would like now to say a bit about the aims we have in working with families. First and foremost, of course, we aim to establish understanding and healthy change in the family constellation which will continue into the future, so that the patient will have a healthier environment to which to return. Put another way, we want the family to keep pace with the patient as he progresses, and to be better than ever before. This, after all, is our goal for the patient too. Second, we aim to have relatives see and know us to be everyday human beings, just as we aim to have patients view us as ordinary mortals. Third, we consciously try to help the relative understand the patient's distortions, so that between them there may be more rational communication, mutual tolerance and sympathy. Fourth, we aim to have the family see treatment as a continuous process so that the patient will be aided with aftercare. Fifth, we strive to help the relative overcome the prejudices and suspicions about psychiatry to which he is subject in our culture. Essentially, I suppose, we aim for the relative to develop faith in psychiatrists as people. This seems to be particularly necessary when relatives have been bitter for having been excluded from the ambulatory treatment-situation. The relative who asks, "Why didn't the doctor see me or tell me when things were so bad? I wanted to see him but he was too busy," is expressing a general resentment toward psychiatrists. Remarks such as these, heard often enough, alerted us to see relatives regularly if we wished their cooperation.

Additionally, I believe that in working with families we are trying to have the relative "sympathize" with us—to appreciate the difficulty and complexity of our task. We acknowledge the relative's share of responsibility in the outcome of treatment. If he fulfills it he may have the personal satisfaction of knowing he contributed to the patient's improvement.

Family therapy is not incidental to the patient's treatment, but essential to it, and an integral part of the patient's whole treatment program. The techniques of its application are as varied as they are in individual therapy. They have been suggested in much of the foregoing, but may be elaborated upon at this point.

There is no well-defined, systematized method of family treatment. Grotjahn says, "The best way of treatment must emerge before the inner eye of the experienced therapist." He adds, therefore, that the best guide for all decisions regarding technique "will always be the patient's or the family's resistance, and the chance the interview will offer to interpret this resistance." I would say that fundamentally I agree with this statement of the case. It does two things: first, it gives us the widest latitude in the application of techniques of accomplishing family therapy; and second, it essentially preserves and leaves room for the use of basic psychoanalytic principles having to do with resistance, transference, counter transference and insight.

Anyone familiar with psychoanalytic practice and principle, therefore, will appreciate that one may see the primary patient with any one or all members of his family, depending on the judgment of the therapist, and as frequently as decided by the therapist. The way the therapist is to conduct himself will also be his decision, dependent on the conditions of the moment, and naturally his aim to furnish insight to one and all. I will suggest, however, that family therapy is not the field of endeavor for the inexperienced or rash therapist, but, as Grotjahn says, for the one who can be "as free, as spontaneous, as honest and frank" as he can be. To this I might add that the therapist should be as objective, as brave, without being foolhardy, and as partial, when certain he is free of countertransference taint, as he may be.

The family therapist cannot be too protective of his primary patient, for in reality the entire family is his patient. He should be ready to saddle his patient, whenever it is true, with responsibility for any particular unhealthy condition in the family. He should not be too bound by psychoanalytic tradition, as regards both principle and technique, because he is navigating uncharted waters. He must, therefore, be a creative experimenter, and free to see new principles, no matter how personally threatening they may seem, and to seize opportunities for new techniques.

At the very least, the family therapist must be prepared to be very active in the treatment situation, and to shift his emphasis from the interpretation of the unconscious toward analysis of resistances and toward the integration of the ego. He must be prepared to deal less with the transference situation on a verbal level, and more with the current interactional, rather than intrapsychic, sphere. In treating a family we ourselves are not loathe to manage, direct, and suggest—to "structure" the situation by taking a commanding role. This is done on the basis of our interpretations of events or interactions we observe within the family. We may verbalize these interpretations or not. Family therapy also calls for a certain amount of education of the relative into the intricacies of the patient's mind. Family members must be helped to see how a patient may misinterpret their behavior, no matter how reasonable it may appear to them. We, therefore, interpret their behavior for them and help them to see how it *actually* affects the patient, as opposed to the way they intend it to.

During the past decade we have dealt with the significant family members of some seven hundred and fifty inpatients. Quite early in this experience we saw the undeniable value the family could have in the patient's treatment program. It took but a short time for us to develop a sympathetic attitude toward the patient's family, and to expand the number and the nature of our contacts with it. Perhaps, since we spent a great deal of "living time" with our patients in our intensive treatment-atmosphere, our "sympathetic attitude" really became a "bond of sympathy" which arose out of our growing appreciation of the problems the family must have had in living with the patient. This may have led us, initially, to try merely to relieve the family's anxiety and distress. It did not take long to see, however, that these sessions with the family had a therapeutic effect as evidenced by healthy changes in these people. Naturally, we were encouraged to increase the number, regularity and quality of these contacts.

Experience taught us that our relationship to the primary patient was not jeopardized, and, if anything, the patient encouraged us to convey certain "secrets" to the relative that he was not as yet brave enough to disclose directly. We found that as our therapeutic community atmosphere developed we were telling relatives how their patient was relating as a human being with other patients—rather than what their gross symptoms were. This turned out to be quite similar to the way the patient had related to the relative, and fruitful discussions then followed about internal family problems. Naturally, as these talks became more personal, emotional crises arose which were similar to those which we were learning had also arisen between the patient and the relative. It didn't take much more for us to see that we should at times bring patient and relative together, particularly when our best efforts with each individually were to no avail. It is quite common for us consciously to take a therapeutic approach to family members seen individually, an approach designed to fit into the patient's current therapeutic status.

We believe that in working with families therapeutically we achieve the aims mentioned earlier in this paper. Not only have we seen patients change for the better characterologically, but also families, and have attributed this to the nature of our work with them as a family unit. I believe I can say that given a fair therapeutic risk, and ample time, we never accomplish a good therapeutic result without simultaneously achieving a positive change in the family, or some significant member of it.

I would not want to leave any impression that the task is easy, but experience enables one to handle families with increasing ease. The process, however, is a time-consuming one, and requires a highly integrated hospital organization, with a medical staff that has ample time for it. Additionally, the therapists must fully accept the approach as valuable to their respective patients, not one they follow under compulsion.

Family therapy has enormous value. I know that it has enabled us to help certain patients with whom we otherwise would have failed. I don't know now how we could go about treating patients without therapeutic attention to the family. As a matter of fact, we feel handicapped in treating a patient with no readily available relative. In this event particularly we find ourselves studying the manner in which patients relate to staff as surrogate figures. To a large extent in our therapeutic community atmosphere we tend to regard our small group of patients and personnel as something of a family group.

Family therapy gives us a quicker and incomparably deeper understanding of the patient's psychopathology. It also makes the latter's origins clearer to us. Family therapy enables us actively to help more people, and to ensure a better prognosis for the patient insofar as he returns to a healthier family. From the research point of view it offers psychiatry an opportunity to learn more about human psychopathology and the techniques of its treatment. In some respects we may regard or develop family therapy as a research tool (for certainly it is not easy to utilize in everyday practice), a tool which furnishes us answers to otherwise insoluble problems. As an addition to our armamentarium it can diminish the frequency with which we are frustrated in psychiatry. At the very least, if it gives us additional hope it has great value. Who of us long in the practice of psychiatry, particularly with psychotic patients, has not felt the need of more hope?

There are a number of open questions which might be indicated at this point. All of them would seem in need of our consideration and exploration in psychiatry. As yet we have no definite idea of the type of family that can benefit from family therapy, let alone the nature of the end result we would seek for it. I am sure that with time we will be able to determine the type of family pathology which will respond to our efforts, and which will not. In the inpatient setting, too, we have yet to learn which family member should be treated by the primary patient's therapist, and which might have to have a collaborating therapist. The primary patient's role and effect on both therapist and family member is a subject in itself in this context.

Family treatment seems to have a logical relationship to the therapeutic community concept. It is likely that with time we will witness the family taking an increasing role in the hospital care of the inpatient. Evidences of this are already present. How this might be worked out in a helpful way needs to be discovered and described. Additionally, we could benefit from more extensive investigation of the effects family therapy actually has on the family as a unit, as well as on its members as individuals. As yet our understanding along these lines is admittedly superficial. All we can be quite certain of is that the technique of family therapy is beneficial to those concerned. Finding the methods involved useful, we may be encouraged to apply them to individual therapy, particularly with the difficult schizophrenic.

The point has been made that in family therapy one may study current interaction and produce healthy change without resorting to a study of libidinal drives and "origins" of pathology. The suggestion, therefore, is that one may in this way build on the patient's healthy attributes without helping him to know "why" he got sick in the first place—if indeed the early traumatic events we now believe to be causative are really so, and, more particularly, the "insight" we furnish is really the causative factor in producing health. We may consider the point that the patient may recover from illness without knowing "why" he got sick, just as one may be "healthy" in the first place without knowing why he developed so.

REFERENCES

1. Oberndorf, C. P.: *Folie à Deux*. Int. J. Psychoanal., 15: 14-24, 1934.
2. Mittelman, B.: *Complementary Neurotic Reactions in Intimate Relationships. Psychoanal. Quart.*, 13: 479-491, 1944.
3. ——: *The Concurrent Analysis of Married Couples. Ibid.*, 17: 182-197. 1948.
4. ——: "Simultaneous Treatment of Both Parents and Their Children," in *Specialized Techniques of Psychotherapy* (G. Bychowski and J. L. Despert, Eds.). New York: Basic Books, 1952.
5. Martin, P. A. and H. W. Bird: *An Approach to the Psychotherapy of Marriage Partners*. Psychiatry, 16: 123-127, 1953.
6. Thomas, A.: *Simultaneous Psychotherapy with Marital Partners*. Am. J. Psychother., 10: 716-727, 1956.
7. Ackerman, N. W. *The Psychodynamics of Family Life*. New York: Basic Books, 1958.
8. Jackson, D. D.: "Family Interaction, Family Homeostasis and Some Implications for the Conjoint Family Psychotherapy," in *Individual and Familial Dynamics* (Jules H. Masserman, Ed.). New York: Grune & Stratton, 1959.
9. Grotjahn, M.: *Psychoanalysis and the Family Neurosis*. New York: Norton, 1960.

11

Conjoint Family Therapy in the Inpatient Setting

EDWIN L. RABINER, M.D.
HANS MOLINSKI, M.D.
ALEXANDER GRALNICK, M.D.

INTRODUCTION

In recent years the subject and practice of family therapy has commanded increasing attention in psychiatry. The major work thus far has been done in the field of research with families placed in a hospital setting, together with the primary patient,[1] or with ambulatory patients and their families.[2] In most instances primary patients have been children or adolescents. In addition a number of papers have been devoted to efforts directed at understanding[3] and treating the relatives of inpatients in order to aid the therapeutic task with the primary patient and to make his future life with them more tolerable.[4,5,6]

Little work has been reported concerning treatment by joint interview of members of the family together with the psychotic inpatient. The present paper is a preliminary report of our experience with this conjoint* family therapy approach in the inpatient setting. To some extent it is the logical evolution both of some of our former work and the nature of our treatment facilities already described in previous pa-

Reprinted from *American Journal of Psychotherapy,* Vol. XVI, No. 4, pp. 618-631. October, 1962.

* The term conjoint is borrowed from Jackson. [7,8]

pers.[9,10] Primary patients in our series range in age from adolescence to the sixties.

I. Family Involvement in the Inpatient Treatment Process

It is increasingly accepted that one cannot hope to do too well with the psychotic, particularly schizophrenic, inpatient with the aid of the one-to-one psychotherapeutic relationship alone, analytically oriented or otherwise. Schizophrenia is an isolating process that destroys the patient's judgment and makes him a trial to others. It is a crippling disease which frustrates and exhausts the best of therapists who attempt its resolution purely on their own. Those who would adjust to and help the schizophrenic must therefore care for him a great deal. As such the family unit, often made up of the very individuals who have abetted the schizophrenic's retreat from reality, has a vital role to play. The family's empathic support or lack of it through the long, costly, and trying treatment process crucially affects its outcome. Failure to acknowledge this has, perhaps, all too often led us to rely upon the one-to-one psychotherapeutic relationship, only to find that our own stores of love, understanding, and personal ministrations are inadequate to the task, especially since our own families have prior claim to them.

It is a striking fact that when one immerses himself in the treatment of psychotic inpatients and sees their family members frequently, one develops feelings of sympathy for the family. This is not to say that less positive attitudes do not also present themselves. Usually, however, one does find oneself assuming responsibility for the welfare of family members as well as for the patient. It is likely that this "countertransference phenomenon," if it may be called that, has been an important motor force in the evolution of family therapy. It is clear that changes in the primary patient, along with decisions one makes for him or helps him make for himself, impinge upon the family group with effects one must take into account.

The major task of the inpatient center is to bring the patient to a level permitting return to the community or family for further ambulatory care. Put another way, pathology must be reduced or circumscribed to a point that makes life in extramural society feasible. For the schizophrenic, with his social mobility frozen by his pathology, this means making life in the biologic family unit feasible.

Central to our own quest of this goal has been the planned replication in the inpatient setting of specific structural elements and interactional demands characteristic of family life. In this regard fellow-patients and hospital personnel are viewed as surrogate family members. The patient lives in a new, therapeutically controlled social field upon which family conflicts are replayed. His life experience in it, as well as the psychotherapeutic utilization of observations of his life style in relation to it, have, we feel, contributed significantly to our effectiveness in achieving this major task.

All too often, however, we have seen hard won gains in relation to the "intramural family" dissipate themselves toward the end of hospitalization as they are tested against increasing exposure to the vicissitudes of life in the untreated family to which the patient must return. In effect, in many instances, it has appeared insufficient to attempt to create within the inpatient setting an environment patterned on healthy family interaction conducive to individual growth and repair without extending these efforts into the actual family unit.

Other factors derived from the extent of the schizophrenic's interpersonal disability further substantiate the importance of intensive work with the families of such patients. We know that there is a universal tendency in the human personality to persevere in wresting from its primary frustrators a greater measure of gratification. Whether conceptualized in the context of Freud's "repetition compulsion" or Silverberg's concept of "transference",[11] every individual seeks to recreate unsatisfactory situations in order to resolve them better. For the personality sufficiently intact to form new relationships, the potential exists for repair of self-esteem in the new relationships. For many schizophrenics, however, the old battles must be fought on the same battleground with the same frustrators. In the face of this, the schizophrenic's helplessness to alter family members' response toward him gives rise to profound despair. If this despair is to be mitigated, the patient needs an active ally to shift the balance of power. When he works in isolation with the patient, the therapist's chances of shifting the tide of battle are perhaps no better than those of the manager in the corner of the outclassed boxer.

The concept of schizophrenic regression which has led to the equating of the schizophrenic and the child has been criticized for reasons having to do with the differences between the two. Yet there is a striking similarity in the helplessness of both to communicate feelings directly rather than by acting out in a fashion that is incomprehensible to family members and merely serves to alienate them.

In the therapy of children in a similar plight, therapists have long since responded to needs implicit in the situation for (1) active intervention to shift the balance of power away from the omnipotent parent, and (2) facilitation of communication between patient and family. In the parallel therapy of children and their parents, the therapist plays both roles, setting limits for parents and interpreting to them the meaning of the primary patient's behavioral communications. In the treatment of adults, however, we have tended to avoid the contamination of the relationship that might result from direct contact between therapist and family members. For the schizophrenic inpatient this sacrosanct position of the one-to-one psychotherapeutic relationship seems hardly justified by the results achieved with it, especially since it blocks a frontal approach to the problem of the schizophrenic's obligatory dependency upon family members who need help in adequately responding. That degree of accommodation to family members, therefore, which the patient cannot make despite our best treatment efforts, requires direct intervention in the family situation.

To date such intervention on the part of inpatient centers has taken the following forms: (1) Casework interview, usually by someone other than the therapist of the primary patient; (2) referral for psychotherapy, usually to a therapist having little or no contact with the treatment center; (3) parallel interview of family members by the therapist of the primary patient.

Conjoint family therapy as a fourth technique of family intervention seems to us most specifically addressed to the assessment and alteration of family interaction. Thus it minimizes the misperceptions implicit in the second-hand reporting of family transactions. It avoids the interposition of an additional relay station (caseworker or other therapist) with its possibilities of introducing further distortion and widening the gulf. It affords the therapist the greatest opportunity to observe and confront the family with its interactional distortions.

II. The Conjoint Family Process

A number of workers with a variety of theoretical orientations have written on this subject. Common to all these orientations has been the primary aim of structuring the interview situation so as to encourage a maximum interplay between family members, with the therapist serving (1) to decode veiled communications, and (2) to provide role clarification for the involved family members while protecting the participating individuals against joint assault through the transient shifting of his support as the process unfolds. In this setting the aim is to foster a feeling of cooperative effort toward more gratifying family life, to clarify the mutual needs and expectations of each family member, to explore the self-defeating ways in which these needs are currently being sought and to elucidate, wherever possible, the historical determinants of individual patterns of self-defeat, making the provocative behavior of each more comprehensible to the other until it can be beneficially altered.

III. Tactical Advantages in the Inpatient Setting

It is a common experience to find that in precisely those instances where the need to alter family members' pathology is most crucial to the outcome of therapy with the primary patient, the severity of pathology either makes the family member refractory to treatment referral or precipitates acting out. Guilt feelings about having brought the patient to the hospital, and about having contributed to the primary patient's illness, are often intensified by a direct treatment recommendation to the family member. This may lead to a family member's acting out so as to sabotage the primary patient's treatment opportunity. On the other hand, the proposal on the patient's behalf of joint meetings of the family with the patient and therapist is far less likely to arouse defensiveness. Under the face-saving illusion of being a "co-therapist" (which will be dealt with later in the conjoint therapy) we have found family members to be generally enthusiastic in their response to this proposal. Furthermore, inclusion in the patient's active treatment tangibly conveys to the family members an appreciation of their true significance in the patient's life and prospects. This feeling of inclusion reinforces positive and constructive motivations in the family member. It contrasts with the guilt reinforcing effect frequently seen to result from the traditional practice of barring active participation of the family in the treatment effort.

Frequently, the schizophrenic patient in his great anxiety at being hospitalized, cut off from symbiotic gratification, fearful of losing what little social identity he may have possessed, and convinced that things cannot be changed anyway, sees no other way open to him but illness. This circumstance manifests itself as "a lack of motivation," seemingly "insurmountable defensiveness" and "bad judgment." He wants nothing but release from the hospital without regard to whether he is ready or not. He may be assisted in his wish by the family's own needs. At times the relative's needs may be even more instrumental to an untimely departure than his own tremendous anxiety and hopelessness. This "lack of motivation" so typical of him, or lack of objectivity, or both, so typical of his family, tends to deprive him of the treatment that is available. The schizophrenic often needs the firm guidance of his family who should not permit him to bolt from treatment. Clearly the need for prompt engagement of the family in rehabilitative efforts is of vital importance in establishing and maintaining the treatment situation. In this regard the conjoint setting offers families a number of constructive opportunities in addition to evidence from us of their importance to the patient's prospects, and the guilt mollifying feeling of participation. First, it affords the family access to the patient under carefully controlled circumstances at a time when unsupervised contacts might lead to further injury to the patient and reciprocal acting out by family and patient. Furthermore, patent manifestations of the patient's continuing pathology can be either directly observed by them or subsequently elucidated by the therapist. Distortions feeding their mutual anxieties can be minimized and promptly dealt with since all data are directly available to all participants, including the therapist. Direct witnessing of the therapist's competence and interest in the family do much to foster positive attitudes on the part of the family toward the inpatient center.

Conjoint family therapy also provides important tactical advantages for the patient. Feelings of isolation from the family are mitigated by the frequent contacts with them which might be contraindicated for him if unsupervised. Of great importance, we think, is the contribution such meetings can make toward mitigating the pervasive sense of hopelessness described above. Because the schizophrenic process results in withdrawal from reality bound, constructive efforts to deal with overwhelming interpersonal anxieties, primarily involving family figures who remain everlastingly important, it creates an abiding sense of hopelessness. In our view this often limits development of the psychotherapeutic relationship with the schizophrenic, who in effect says, "I need to believe that if I give the world a second chance things will be better for me. In the absence of evidence of this I will cling to my illness for what little comfort it affords me." In the face of such hopelessness, some therapists have devoted years of their time to attempts at proving via sustained accepting relationships with patients that the world deserves a second chance.

We have seen, in instances like the case illustrations below, a dramatic melting of this frozen hopelessness come about after a series of conjoint therapy sessions. We have attributed this to the following factors:

1. "If the therapist dares to stand up to the omnipotent parent perhaps he or she is less formidable than I believed."

2. "If the therapist can make him or her understand me perhaps I can too," and conversely, "if the therapist cannot understand (that is, double bind) no wonder I can't."

3. "If he or she (family member) can accept, without falling apart or viciously retaliating, the therapist's criticism (confrontations, interpretations) then maybe I, too, can risk self-assertion."

4. Spontaneous remarks by relatives, for example, "I never looked at it that way before," as well as shifts in family alliances, no matter how transient, create the impression that change is possible.

Further unique potentialities of the conjoint treatment setting work to the advantage of the treatment staff. In the inpatient setting, one is often confronted with the difficult task of having to help a patient decide between moving toward or moving away from family members. Prognosis for sustaining even a marginal extramural existence, as well as for further growth, is often directly contingent upon the family's ability to accept changes in the patient and to alter its attitudes and interactional patterns in response to these changes. Traditionally, the impact upon the patient of increasing exposure to family members toward the end of a hospitalization has been the sole means of prognostically assaying these factors. All too often, by the time trouble signs appear on visits, the patient or his family, or both, have taken the bit in their teeth and consider the patient to be on convalescent status, so that the opportunity for further work is lost. We have found conjoint family therapy to provide an excellent predictive basis with regard to the stresses to which return to the family setting will expose the patient. Since this information can be gathered in an exclusively intramural hospital setting as a part of treatment, rather than on weekend visits as a part of convalescent extramural reintegration into family life, the reins are more likely to remain in the therapist's hands.

Thus far we have spoken primarily of the potentialities of the conjoint family treatment situation for solidly establishing and maintaining the treatment situation of the primary inpatient. Perhaps of even greater significance are its potentialities for the "long pull," the total rehabilitative program.

The needs and expectations of patient and family members of each other can be interpreted in parallel interviews. The conjoint setting, however, has the decisive advantage of having all the raw data of aberrant communication and perception vividly available to all participants. Under these circumstances the therapist's decoding of ambivalent and veiled communication becomes a potent generator of insight, especially since the involved parties are present to confirm dramatically such translations. Several examples of this phenomenon are given below.

CASE HISTORIES

Case 1. J. R., a 21-year-old, single schizophrenic girl had lived in a symbiotic relationship to her mother, which isolated both of them from the father and sister. The father and sister had simply resigned themselves to their exclusion, playing along in their helplessness to change it, in order to get what little gratification they could from both of them. Typical of this symbiosis was the patient's custom, upon returning home after a date, of getting into bed with her mother, to the father's chagrin, and recounting the most intimate details of the evening. The patient's gratification in this symbiosis existed alongside of the simultaneous protestation that mother violated her privacy and would not let her grow up.

Progress made in the patient's individual psychotherapy was repeatedly vitiated by the mother's coercive maneuvers in response to the patient's efforts to maintain a separate identity. The therapists' repeated attempts in parallel interviews over a six-month period failed completely to bring to the mother's awareness the nature of her growth restricting activity. On several occasions these attempts were followed by calls from the father pressuring for the patient's early discharge.

During the fourth conjoint session (thirteenth hospital month), in relation to a question about expressing her feelings to her parents, the patient said, "My mother speaks to me as if I were one of her friends." The mother smiled and seemed pleased. Aware of the veiled meaning of this communication, the therapist said, "J. means to say that you treat her as a contemporary and not as a daughter, which is confusing and upsetting to her." With this the patient beamed her approval at the therapist. The father brought confirmatory material and, for the first time, in response to this momentary weakening of the alliance, expressed his feeling of being left out. The mother began to sense currents of deeper meaning in her relationship to her daughter and for the first time realized the implications of the many previous confrontations attempted by the therapist in his one-to-one interviews with her.

Case 2. P. L., a 29-year-old single male schizophrenic, utilizing obsessive-compulsive defensive maneuvers to control otherwise unmanageable angry feelings toward others for perceived slights, was seen in joint interview with his mother after lengthy preparation via parallel sessions. She asked, "Do you want to see me next visiting day?" The therapist knew that he wanted to see her and was angry that she did not put her wish to see him in more affirmative terms. He also knew that she desperately wished to see the patient but wanted some prior commitment from the patient lest she go too far out on the proverbial limb. The patient was about to react violently to her question which he experienced as another rejection of him.

Rather than risk letting them go on to work it out with much heat and some risk of their being driven further apart, the therapist elucidated these dynamics, bringing dramatic awareness of the similar fear of rejection underlying their mutual response to each other.

In our experience, the process of decoding of communication, initially performed primarily by the therapist, rarely fails to excite the interest of all participants, motivating them toward more conscious efforts to decode for themselves. In effect, the conjoint treatment process provides a valuable educative or retraining experience which, in time, makes it decreasingly necessary for a therapist to serve as a communication bridge. Where family members are reasonably pliable, this experience of "really listening" and communicating more directly may suffice to turn the tide in favor of the patient's continued extramural adjustment following discharge.

Often, however, it is necessary to regard the family's conjoint treatment experience in the hospital as the first step in their ongoing treatment which needs to continue following discharge of the primary patient. In such instances we have seen the hospital family treatment experience serve in good stead in overcoming resistances of family members to an ongoing treatment situation for them. The following case is illustrative of such a result.

Case 3. S., a 22-year-old relapsing catatonic schizophrenic whose hospitalization was precipitated by an attempt to move away from her psychotic family through attendance at an out-of-town college, had devoted her whole life to magical maneuvers designed to lift mother and brother from psychosis under the grandiose, dependency denying delusion that she alone could save them. At the same time she felt a painful loss of personal identity in her dedication to save them, and hated her mother for being enslaved by her. It became clear during her hospitalization that the extent of her ego disability precluded in the foreseeable future a life independent of her family, leaving only chronic hospitalization as an alternative to returning to this destructive family field. Although the patient's father had for many years been in psychotherapy for recurrent depressions, the mother had stubbornly resisted all efforts to get her to seek help despite the fact that for ten years she had urged her withdrawn schizophrenic son to enter therapy. The father died during the patient's hospitalization. Thereafter, mother and son were constantly at each other's throats over the management of the apartment house left to them by the father. A further complication, when the hospital staff contemplated the patient's return home, lay in her continued erotic feelings for her brother. There had been overt sexual encounters between the patient and her brother subsequent to which they had completely ignored and avoided each other.

During the eighth hospital month, after attempts to get mother and brother into therapy had failed, conjoint family therapy "to help the patient" was begun on a once-a-week basis. The patient was seen twice weekly by the therapist in the intervals between the joint interviews. During the ensuing four months, the mother's need, heightened by her husband's death, to snatch the patient from the hospital for her own symbiotic gratification was controlled. The patient and her brother began to communicate again. The initial screaming at each other by mother and brother gave way to more controlled and meaningful communication under the therapist's steadying influence. The mother began for the first time to make such spontaneous statements as "maybe it isn't so good for S. to sleep in my bedroom." The patient gained the courage to assert tentatively her individuality to her mother, and began to feel that saving her mother was a burden shared by the therapist and therefore not exclusively hers. The possibility that something could be done about their long frozen despair with each other gave new hope to all three. Family tensions, though far from resolved, diminished to a point that made the patient's discharge feasible. All three enthusiastically accepted a referral for ambulatory family therapy.

IV. Preparation for Conjoint Family Therapy in the Inpatient Setting

Some of the considerations entering into the selection of cases for conjoint family therapy have already been alluded to. Actually, we find ourselves hard put to state categorically a set of indications for its use. We consider it to be indicated, at least on a trial basis, when:

1. Current or anticipated tensions between patient and family significantly affect the patient's intramural or potential extramural adjustment.

2. We have gained a sufficient knowledge of the strengths and weaknesses of the primary patient and family members to form judgments in the following areas:

(a) The defensive necessities underlying the role played by each member of the family are not so fixed and desperate as to lead to decompensation upon conjoint exploration of them.

(b) There exist unfulfilled mutual needs of family members and patient to relate to each other in a more gratifying way.

(c) The reactions of all parties to the initial stress of joint family interview within predictable limits will be manageable by the therapist in his supportive and protective role toward each.

(d) The primary patient has developed a sufficient positive transference to the therapist so that inquiry into the determinants of his own behavior in the joint setting is possible without jeopardizing the existing rapport between patient and therapist.

3. The involved family members can arrange to come to the hospital at least once a week.

Having on these grounds decided to attempt conjoint family therapy, we have pursued the following procedure. The therapist waits for an appropriate cue, such as the patient's mention of some feeling about a situation that has transpired with family members during a visit or phone call which reflects a communication disturbance between the parties involved. He suggests to the patient that communication problems such as this might be resolved by frank discussion between the parties involved in the presence of the therapist. If the patient seems willing and not unduly anxious at the prospect, the therapist sees the family, elicits their impressions and feelings about the particular exchange and presents the patient's point of view. Several interviews may be necessary before the patient is brought in. Should the patient seem unduly fearful about such a meeting, this fear is specifically examined in individual psychotherapy until, assured of the therapist's support, and aware of the irrational determinants of the fear, the patient seems willing.

The joint session is arranged and enjoined by the therapist in the following fashion. "We've arranged to get together here to see if frank discussion of some of your feelings about each other can be helpful to you. As I've explained to you individually, such discussion is not easy. It can be most helpful, however, if you can try to listen and feel along with each other as you talk, although we all have a tendency to be most open to our own feelings and viewpoints. It might be well to begin with the recent incident that we've discussed individually."

Thus having launched conjoint family therapy, the therapist begins his role in it as interpreter, arbiter, and protector, pointing out in the early phases evidence of problems in empathy and meaningful communication between the parties as they unfold. Conjoint interviews are held on a once-a-week basis. The primary patient is seen twice-a-week and transactions of the joint interview, with particular emphasis on the patient's contributions, are minutely discussed. Analogous reactions in the patient's "intramural family" process are mustered by the therapist in studying with the patient his role in the conjoint setting. Family members are seen without the patient, when indicated, between successive joint interviews. Joint interviews may be temporarily abandoned when they appear too stressful for the parties involved, to be resumed after further individual interviews have resolved the intercurrent crisis.

V. Goals of Conjoint Family Therapy in the Inpatient Setting

We have already described some of the partial aims one may seek with this technique in the inpatient rehabilitative setting in contrast to other practices of family therapy which may deal more totally with reconstructive phenomena. In general, such goals are broadly divisible into five categories:

A. Preserving the patient's treatment opportunity.

B. Improving the conditions for the primary patient's hospital treatment.

C. Facilitating family acceptance of long range treatment goals along with such environmental alterations as may be expedient for the primary patient. This may include treatment placement for family members.

D. The synergistic use of the biologic and intramural family process for the working through of the primary patient's salient patterns of self-defeat.

E. Favorably altering family communication patterns where the patient's post-discharge residence with the family is either mandatory or expedient so that further treatment on an outpatient basis becomes feasible.

Which one or combination of goals is appropriate must, of course, be individually determined. These goals run the gamut from mere environmental manipulation and education to reconstruction of communication and family interaction patterns, and at another level from repressive to uncovering. Just as in individual psychotherapy, where personality reconstruction, though always desirable, is not always feasible, so too, achieving goals in categories D and E though probably conducive to the best prognosis is not always attainable or appropriate to the inpatient setting, when this setting is viewed as a locus for only a part of the total treatment process.

VI. Technical Problems

In our thinking and discussions about the conjoint family process in the inpatient setting much interest centered on the management of the therapists' countertransference. In their high degree of commitment to family therapy, our therapists mirrored those described by Jackson and Weakland,[8] lending further credence to their notion that once one tries it, one is "hooked." Because it works? Perhaps. But this can be tested only by valid outcome studies for which adequate controls would be hard to devise. There is, however, also room to believe that therapists' enthusiasm for this technique may have countertransference determinants. Surely there are few situations that lend themselves more readily to exploitation by the therapists' grandiose strivings. In contrast to the one-to-one psychotherapy model, the therapist must be active. He is forced to regulate verbal traffic in the context of his own value judgments as to what kinds of contributions and by whom will best serve the interests of the process. He is inexorably cast in the role of arbiter, mediator, and judge, carrying the hopes of all participants for acceptance and corroboration under circumstances where the vested interests of all may conflict. The investment of each in these conflicting interests is by virtue of the long history of prior relatedness and conflict between family members far greater than that with which the group therapist must work.

The therapist is apt to see the primary patient as his chief responsibility. Yet it is unlikely that in all cases the primary patient's need for the therapist's support will exceed that of other family members. To whatever extent the therapist carries into the conjoint situation from the one-to-one treatment frame of reference loyalty to the patient rather than to the family unit, he runs the risk of jeopardizing all treatment goals. He must fight a continuing battle against antipathy toward family members who "have brought this suffering upon my patient." He must avoid responding to multiple seductions as well as those inherent in his own omnipotent strivings which constantly beckon him to bludgeon refractory participants into change and compliance with his own notions of how the process should proceed. He must avoid subtly coercing the primary patient in his individual sessions with him to exclude other areas of his total day-today experience for the sake of exalting the therapist's skill in managing family members during conjoint sessions. He must avoid inconsistencies in his attitudes toward the individuals involved as he moves from the conjoint situation to parallel meetings with them. He must avoid countertransference behavior deriving from his own unresolved family problems.

The conjoint situation is highly charged for all its participants. Its high life proximity reduces tolerance for error. And yet the likelihood of countertransference errors of commission is geometrically increased over individual psychotherapy or parallel treatment where the therapist may wear different cloaks in his separate roles with the various individuals involved.

Because the stakes are high and the risk considerable, the decision to employ conjoint interviews is a crucial one, demanding keen clinical judgment on the part of the therapist. On several occasions we have seen the enthusiasm of therapists for this procedure compromise their clinical judgment, leading to an antitherapeutic reestablishment of symbiotic ties or disturbances of the therapists' rapport with the primary patient, or both. To avoid such unfavorable results, it is of paramount importance that (1) the therapist be fully aware of his own motivations in recommending this procedure, and (2) the primary patient and family members be adequately prepared for it.

SUMMARY

The critical importance of involving family members in the inpatient treatment of schizophrenia has been discussed in the light of the obligatory dependence of the schizophrenic upon his family as well as of the situationally determined needs of both. Special adaptation of conjoint family therapy practice as well as its particular advantages in the inpatient setting have been described along with case illustrations. The synergistic use of conjoint family interview process and the intramural "social-family process" appears, at least to the authors, to merit further investigation and replication in order to enhance our therapeutic effectiveness with the schizophrenic inpatient.

REFERENCES

1. Bowen, M.: The Family as the Unit of Study and Treatment. *Am. J. Orthopsychiat.* 31: 1, 1961.
2. Ackerman, N. and Behrens, M.: The Family Group and Family Therapy. In *Progress in Psychotherapy.* Grune & Stratton, New York, 1958.
3. Gralnick, A.: The Carrington Family—A Psychiatric and Social Study Illustrating the Psychosis of Association or Folie à Deux. *Psychiat. Quart.* 17: 2, 1943.
4. Lefebvre, P. et al: The Role of the Relative in a Psychotherapeutic Program. *J. Canad. Psychiat. Assoc.* 3: 110, 1958.
5. Gralnick, A.: The Family in Psychotherapy. In *Individual and Familial Dynamics.* J. Masserman, Ed., Grune & Stratton, New York, 1959.
6. Gralnick, A.: Relation of the Family to a Psychotherapeutic Inpatient Program. *Int. J. Soc. Psychiat.* 5: 131, 1959.
7. Jackson, D.: Family Interaction, Homeostasis and some Implications for Conjoint Family Psychotherapy. In *Individual and Familial Dynamics.* J. Masserman, Ed., Grune & Stratton, New York, 1959.
8. Jackson, D. and Weakland, J. Conjoint Family Therapy. *Psychiatry,* 24: 2 (Supplement), 1961.
9. Gralnick, A. and D'Elia, F.: Role of the Patient in Therapeutic Community: Patient-Participation. *Am. J. Psychother.,* 15: 63, 1961.
10. Gralnick, A.: Family Psychotherapy. General and Specific Consideration. *Am. J. Orthopsychiat.* 32:3, 1962.
11. Silverberg, W. V.: *Childhood Experience and Personal Destiny: A Psychoanalytic Theory of Neurosis.* Springer Publ. Co., New York, 1952.

12
Family Therapy

ALEXANDER GRALNICK, M.D.
PETER H. SCHWEEN, M.D.

THE TRADITIONAL general practitioner may be looked upon as the forerunner of the present-day psychiatric family-therapist. His role was that of father figure, counselor, advisor, and omnipotent being possessed of an uncanny understanding of the individual as well as of the family group. He was cast, or cast himself, as the being with better knowledge not only of the physical aspects of life, but also of its psychological. Comprehension of the physiology of one's emotional life was taken to mean he was better prepared to know its social origins and ultimate effects on the person and those about him. Basically the physician was looked to as the repository of that wisdom of the ages which seemed so necessary to guide the sick and ailing of mind, heart, and body. It was, of course, known that little of this knowledge came from books the doctor studied. It did seem to emanate from experience with people in their most troubled times. This is not to mean that others, such as religious leaders, did not also play significant roles in this regard. However, none commanded this respected position, and played the role as uniformly and universally as did the family doctor.

The manner in which one sets about doing things is often determined by many matters of a fortuitous nature. Often such factors lead to a discovery, or habits, which one in

Reprinted from *Psychiatric Research Report* 20, pp. 212-217, American Psychiatric Association, February 1966.

turn finds most convenient, regardless of ensuing circumstances, and which he then is inclined to describe as the better way of doing things. A situation of this nature had to do with our finally instituting family therapy some ten years ago. When we started High Point Hospital in 1951, budgetary limitations precluded the employment and traditional use of social workers. Medical time was not at a premium, and therefore all contacts between therapists and relatives were direct. The patient's psychiatrist took the original anamnesis, maintained telephonic and subsequent personal contact with the family, and accomplished the usual things intended to allay the relative's anxiety, win his understanding, and direct the nature of his communications with the patient. It seems that from this state of affairs, plus the fact that a psychotherapist will automatically practice his profession, no matter with whom he is speaking, there evolved at our hospital what would seem to be more clearly defined as "family therapy."

We like to believe that as we saw more of relatives and their suffering we responded humanly with an increasing conscious offer of assistance in the only way we knew, namely, psychotherapy. True, as our program developed and we ourselves were exposed intensively to the same "slings and arrows" from the patients with which the relatives themselves had been suffering, perhaps we turned to them for a bit of understanding ourselves. Certainly we detected more practical and concrete reason for sympathizing with the relative. Perhaps as he saw our concern and dilemma there grew something of the bond which often develops between people engaged in a common task. We were unaware of the possibility that matters of a countertransference nature might be operating. At any rate, we did begin to see that not all relatives were "bad," nor were they necessarily the entire, if any cause of the patient's illness. In fact, some seemed more than a bit genuinely concerned, some seemed to have good understanding, and many seemed to be well-intentioned, although perhaps misguided.

Most relatives wanted to be of help and many could be in a variety of ways. All complained that the referring psychiatrist pretty uniformly had not seen them, although they had pleaded to be seen so that they might help. They felt "left out" and that important information they had could, therefore, not be transmitted to the therapist. Such information the patient would not tell the doctor. Things seemed to go from bad to worse, and finally, here was the patient in the hospital. Most of all they felt the psychiatrist to be hostile to them. They had been made to feel guilty, as though they were the perpetrators of the patient's illness. What could they do? It did not seem to them that they were to blame. If anyone was to blame it was the psychiatrist. What did he have against them? Why had he not told them that things were so serious? Here, all of a sudden now, the patient needed to be hospitalized, and they had had not one ounce of warning.

Now this may seem like something of a caricature, but I assure you this was the common story some years ago. In more recent years the situation has changed, undoubtedly due to the acceptance of family therapy. A therapist, even a psychoanalyst, need not be apologetic if he sees his patient's relative, even in a conjoint session. The one-to-one relation is not quite as hallowed, and some matters the patient discusses are less sacrosanct. All of which may be looked upon as reason to believe we have made some progress.

If the nature of one's experience makes him what he ultimately is, so the nature of one's clinical experience determines what the psychiatrist believes and puts into practice. Exposure to the relatives of inpatients teaches one the nature of their emotions ranging from feelings of shame and fears of stigma, to those of guilt and hostility, self-loathing and self-pity. Bewilderment, anxiety, and panic at the prospect of re-establishing the family's homeostatic balance with the permanently traumatized, and traumatizing member are evident. The vision of the family without the emotional support the sick member once was to one or several of its members is frightening. The defensive operations to which relatives will resort are legion. All of these play out in the inpatient psychotherapeutic setting in which the psychiatrist takes an active role with the family, and may be seen as no different from what transpires within the family constellation itself. They are revealing of the dynamics of the particular family, and its psychopathology, and of each individual involved.

Leading exponents of the value of family therapy believe that a sick member exists only in a sick family. Only the latter, they believe, could have given rise to the former. This belief stems in turn from the conception that social experience determines the nature of man, and mainly excludes the hereditary or biochemical origin of mental illness. It arises from a philosophy of life as well as a type of clinical experience, let alone a way of evaluating that experience. Family therapy, then, has an inevitable logic for such thinkers.

In the service of objectivity, however, due weight should be given to the fact that many believe mental illness to be self-determined, either on an hereditary or biochemical basis. They do not hold that the presence of a sick member denotes the fact of a sick family. Instead, they argue, that the sick member upsets an otherwise healthy family. They believe that the patient needs restoration so that the family equilibrium may be re-established. They question the wisdom, let alone the propriety of burdening the others with implicit guilt and responsibility. They warn that compelling the others to "adjust" to the sick member through family therapy is an unfair, back-breaking business which may lower their capacity to function healthily. They question the ethic of helping the sick one at the price of threatening, if not actually destroying the mental health of the other. They do not believe that a sick family spawns the sick person.

Whatever the theoretical arguments for or against the rationale and use of family therapy, our particular clinical experience with inpatients led us to see the value of treating with, and finally treating, the family unit. It only remained to define its purpose, to develop treatment techniques, to determine its indications, to determine its positive as well as negative aspects, to assess the problems it presented, to integrate it into our training program as well as our administrative organization, to weigh its effect on the individual psychotherapy with the patient in question let alone the whole program already based on the primacy of individual psychoanalytically-oriented psychotherapy, to determine its cost in time and money, to explore its effect on the therapist practiced in and oriented to individual therapy, and to determine the therapist's role in this form of therapy as contrasted to that in individual therapy. Otherwise the task was relatively simple.

The short time allotted this presentation will not permit me to discuss all of these facets of family therapy. However, I would like to touch on the indications for its use, the main techniques we use, the role of the therapist in it, and what helpful expansion of our knowledge it offers beyond that gained from individual therapy.

The indications for family therapy simultaneously suggest the nature of the family's psychopathology. I list those which we have learned from our experience with psychotic inpatients and their relatives. *First,* such therapy is indicated in the presence of an impasse in the patient's progress, particularly if it is the result of conflict between him and a family member which they cannot resolve on their own. *Second,* when the patient cannot communicate to the relative significant material which needs to be known for the resolution of intrafamily conflicts, the patient can more easily do so in the presence of his therapist. *Third,* in the presence of obvious symbiotic relationships or other severe pathological interrelationships within the family. *Fourth,* when there is a threat of imminent and obviously premature rupture of marital, or other relationships due to unsound understanding of the situation. Left to his own devices on the outside the relative may rapidly conclude that the solution to his problem is to divorce himself from it. The hospital therapist's responsibility to his patient is to prevent this from happening, at least until there has been thorough discussion and reason prevails. Family therapy can accomplish this. *Fifth,* family therapy is useful in helping relatives see and accept the fact, as well as the degree of the patient's illness, and to desist from judging him morally. *Sixth,* family therapy is indicated when there is a threat to the patient's continued hospitalization and treatment as a consequence of distorted understanding between him and the relative.

It is likely that most, if not all of these indications are also applicable to the ambulatory situation. Before instituting family therapy we ordinarily wait until the acute phase has subsided, and the patient has some grasp of the fact that he is sick and the nature of some of his leading problems. It is also useful to have something of a positive atmosphere established between the therapist and the family as well as the therapist and patient. In their absence the therapist must be prepared for particularly difficult times if he engages the family in treatment. The application of family therapy is costly in both the time and energy and financial considerations involved. Additionally, it requires at least several, rather than two people to meet at a mutually convenient time. If for no other reasons, therefore, it is less applicable than individual therapy. Uncommonly it is the only possibility when the individual patient refuses to be treated alone. As a result, its indications should be known, and those therapists who engage in it should be well-trained and convinced of its value.

The purposes of family-therapy are implicit in the indications already mentioned. Essentially it was designed to achieve better results with the patient under treatment. As we went along we discovered that it could produce a more stable family in which the patient had a better chance to maintain his improvement. Family therapy is now designed to help its participants to achieve "insight," to communicate better, to resolve symbiotic relationships, and permit self-identity within the family group. It aims for the establishment of common values and a communality of goals. Simultaneously it seeks a repair of the patient's distortions of reality and poor judgment without imperiling the objectivity and good judgment of the relative.

It seems to me that family therapy started with these rather modest goals, but has more lately assumed more ambitious objectives. If this is so, it is a reflection of the relative helplessness we yet feel in coping with mental illness. We have taken on the task of also understanding family pathology and curing it. We must now know what a sick family is, and what a healthy family must be like, and this before we are too learned about these characteristics in the individual. We are faced with learning how to treat a whole family at a time when we are yet insecure about our ability to successfully treat an individual.

Bound by our experience thus far with the individual patient we yet think in terms of family dynamics and psychopathology and hold that the mere insight into them leads to reparation. Our tendency is to apply the same thinking and techniques of treatment to the family as to the individual. Let us remember, however, that the generally limited success we have had in alleviating the individual patient's suffering, particularly that of the psychotic, has led us into the area of family therapy. It would seem that if we are to be more successful, a novel if not radically different basic approach and technique of treatment may need to be employed.

In the remaining time I would like to say a bit about the types of family therapy we employ. First, we believe we are doing family therapy when the therapist sees his patient together with one or more family members in conjoint sessions over a period of time. While this is the core of family therapy for us, we are at the same time having the therapist treat the patient in individual sessions. We have either not seen reason for, or we have not been brave enough to discontinue individual therapy in favor of doing only family therapy. It may be of significance that no one appears to have done this yet in an inpatient setting.

We consider that we are yet doing family therapy if the conjoint form of it must be temporarily discontinued for one reason or another, and the patient and relative seen independently until they can be brought together in conjoint sessions once more. While conjoint sessions are progressing we will see the relative independently too, if necessary, just as we uniformly see the patient independently. Lately we have been trying another variation, namely, to have the patient and relative seen conjointly by a second therapist who is quite familiar with the family situation, while the patient is also seen individually by his own therapist. The only point I would make is that it appears to us that variations on the theme may be used as long as the stated purposes remain constant.

I might add that we have found family therapy a useful tool in our armamentarium. We use it constantly as the clinical needs of the patient require. We have advanced our knowledge of patients through its use, and have succeeded in accomplishing better results with certain patients. We have seen patients make additional gains once family therapy is added to their regime of individual treatment. However, we have no research study or statistics with which to prove our case. We believe that patients engaged in family therapy return to a healthier family atmosphere, and therefore have a better chance of surviving, but here again we have no follow-up studies to support our belief.

Family therapy, of course, offers us a challenge we cannot deny. It answers our taste and thirst for more knowledge, and holds forth the promise to lead us out of a relative stalemate. It whets our appetite for research, and gives us the security of appearing, if not being, much more knowledgable. It offers to broaden our horizons as psychiatrists, and to expand and improve our techniques as therapists. Above all it presents the opportunity to be of more assistance to our patients, either singly or as a family group. Could one ask for more?

13

Factors Affecting Family Therapy in the Hospital Setting

PETER H. SCHWEEN, M.D.
ALEXANDER GRALNICK, M.D.

FAMILY THERAPY, widely and enthusiastically employed, is still in its initial stages and without the soundest theoretical foundation. In our search for understanding, we have borrowed ideas from the body of psychoanalytic knowledge based on dyadic relationships, from Bertalanffy's general systems theory, and from the "communication" and "role" therapists. The three classical types of family therapy are (1) collaborative family therapy, practiced when two therapists treat different members of a family separately; (2) concurrent or parallel family therapy, practiced when the same therapist sees different fractions of the family at different times; (3) conjoint family therapy, practiced in group treatment of the nuclear or even the extended family. Recently, various modifications have been made. Research has mainly been concerned with interaction within the family as observed in conjoint sessions with hospitalized or ambulatory families. Under the prevalent conditions of family therapy, the family, the patient, and the therapist belong to one and the same milieu. A different situation ensues when a family member becomes hospitalized. In such a case the hospitalized patient and the therapist belong to one medium (the hospital

Reprinted from *Comprehensive Psychiatry,* Vol. 7, No. 5 (October), 1966. pp. 424-431.

milieu) and the family to another medium (the extramural environment). Welding them is a major task.

The increasing trend in psychotherapeutically oriented hospitals to treat the families of inpatients presents several matters for consideration. It will be the purpose of this paper to discuss some of the factors which affect the practice of family therapy with inpatients.

First, in a hospital family therapy is no independent entity. It is but one among other treatment modalities, such as individual psychotherapy, drug and somatic therapy, milieu therapy, and group therapy. Whenever a variety of treatment modalities are employed simultaneously, the danger exists that, instead of enhancing, they may impede one another.[1] The aim then should be to integrate the different modalities in such fashion that each has an optimal effect, the sum total of which will produce the maximal treatment result. Theoretically this would seem to be facilitated by the fact that each type of therapy has its natural focus on another target: individual therapy on intrapsychic events; group, family, and milieu therapy on interactions between people; and drug therapy on mood, affect, and the psychomotor apparatus. Good communication among the psychiatrists in a dynamically oriented hospital as well as the use of the medical staff as a treatment team, helps to achieve the desired optimal integration of the different treatment modalities.

Second, when a patient is hospitalized, his family is not confronted by the family therapist alone, nor is the therapist confronted by the family unit alone. Both have a third "party" with which to contend—namely, the complex apparatus of the hospital organization itself. The patient, the family, and the therapist have to abide by rules as laid down by the hospital. This is not so for ambulatory family therapy, a situation in which the therapist has more control over factors affecting the treatment. The hospital therapist, however, has to abide by the hospital's customs whether he agrees with them or not. In addition, he has to comply with some decisions made by the medical team with regard to the treatment of his patient.

Following is a short description of the treatment program and organization of High Point Hospital. Although it has been more fully described elsewhere,[2,3] we present it here to indicate the nature of the hospital entity and to clarify what we are attempting to convey.

High Point Hospital is a 45-bed service in which the medical staff of seven full-time psychiatrists carries the greatest weight in determining policies. It acts as one of several departments, all of which are interdependent. The psychiatrists work as a team that makes the major decisions on the treatment, including "management," of each patient and his family. "Administration" is seen as one of the elements constituting therapy. Each therapist is endowed with a certain quantum of administrative power. For treatment, the therapeutic modalities described earlier are employed. As part of the milieu program, there are weekly meetings of patients collaborating in work-oriented "committees" in the framework of the hospital's "patient-participation" program. Each committee meets under the supervision and guidance of a staff psychiatrist to fulfill tasks for the hospital's patient population. The emphasis is on studying and correcting the patient's pathologic behavior as he works in cooperation with others. An additional group system exists in the division of the patient population according to levels of "behavior." Five such groups exist, covering a range from maximum supervision and restriction, with a minimum of demands and responsibility, to little supervision, much freedom, and considerable responsibility and self-control. Accordingly, patients are housed on one "closed" and one "open" floor.

Three individual sessions of psychotherapy per week are given each patient. Each staff psychiatrist has a case load of six to eight patients; the Medical Director has none and his assistant has four. Each psychiatrist has immediate responsibility for the physical and emotional state of his patients. In addition, he is responsible for the remaining patients while "officer of the day" and as a member of the staff which confers on all patients regularly. His membership on the "team" entails an extension of his influence, though his autonomy is somewhat curtailed. He is compensated for this curtailment by the opportunity to use the organization of the entire hospital for his therapeutic ends. The Medical Director is a psychiatrist whose background encompasses long experience in hospital and private psychoanalytic practice, in the use of somatic treatment, in hospital administration, and in teaching. He has a large influence on the total program. The staff psychiatrists also have the support of supervising analysts as well as consultants in every medical specialty. No social worker stands between the therapist and the family, but a social group worker coordinates the "patient-participation" program.[4]

The patients are mainly schizophrenic. Violent and severely deteriorated chronic patients are generally excluded. However, severe neurotics and a number of character disorders are admitted. Our "ideal" treatment goal is to initiate or achieve a personality change and to discharge the patient at a higher level of organization than he possessed "premorbidly."

Thus, the family is confronted with (1) a hospital which is a special social structure with its own philosophy and system of values, and (2) a therapist who is in part accountable to a team of colleagues but who also has other treatment modalities at his command. One of these modalities, the milieu, encompasses these very procedures and policies with which he has to comply. Here, of course, is a situation in which the "resentful" therapist may act out his disagreement with the family through the hospital, and vice versa. This point warrants further thought. Just as all methods of treatment may be integrated into a gestalt, so may the whole of this treatment structure be disintegrated into its components. The impetus for the latter may originate in any of its parts. If the switchboard operator is at odds with the medical staff, she may be less adamant in stemming the demands of relatives on a doctor. He may display a hostility toward the family which was originally meant for the switchboard operator. If Business Office personnel feel that the nursing staff handles the patient or family without "due consideration," they may convey this somehow to the family. Families, like patients, are very quick to recognize rifts in the hospital organization and will labor to widen these for their own needs. Since the patient's doctor remains the most important point of contact between the hospital and the family, his conflicts with aspects of the hospital organization will weigh much heavier and the family will see more opportunity to drive a wedge between him and the hospital.

It is well known that family therapy carries with it an increased occurrence of transference and countertransference phenomena. This is even truer when family therapy is conducted within the organization of a hospital. It is a third point we have to consider. Both the family and the patient develop transferential atitudes toward various aspects, departments, staff members, and patients of the hospital. The objects of these attitudes are not fixed and permanent but are interchangeable. This can be quite confusing for the psychiatrist who practices family therapy in a hospital. Sometimes he is treated by the family or by the patient as the exponent of a certain aspect of the hospital, and sometimes as the secret ally of the family trying to turn him against the hospital. He may respond to it properly, but the danger exists that this situation plays into his own transferential attitudes toward the patient, the family, or the hospital personnel. Boszormenyi-Nagy[5] has pointed out that a patient may have a transferentially distorted perception not only of roles but also of interactional patterns. The family therapist in the hospital may also fall prey to a similar transferential misinterpretation of interactions.

In addition, the therapist may act out certain conflicts he has with individual members of the hospital, conflicts which are not of a transferential nature. The family will facilitate this acting out since it corresponds to their needs of manipulating people in order to feel in control of threatening situations. The therapist may be deaf to important information the family supplies because it could confirm the ideas of a colleague whose criticism he rejects. Also, he may have a narcissistic investment in a particular treatment modality which may cause him to neglect other aspects of the treatment program; for example, preference for individual psychotherapy may cause him to disregard the family. Finally, he may, like the family, displace his criticism of society onto the hospital and unwittingly reinforce the views the family harbors instead of correcting them.

When the family in therapy relates to the hospital as a reflection of society, it may attempt to separate the therapist from the hospital team. Several factors come into play. The therapist is significant to the family since the patient's welfare is seen to depend mainly on him. As such he is also a buffer between the family and the hospital. If he can be drawn into the family's orbit, the family can then cast the hospital in an anonymous role, akin to "society," and vent its hostility upon the "institution." Unless the therapist is alert, he is tempted into this trap, sometimes to win favor in the hope that the family will reward him with a good result. He is particular prey to this tactic if he is trying to solve his own problems in relation to the hospital.

There is a fourth aspect of family therapy in the institutional setting worth discussing. It concerns the general problem of the family with a sick member for whom society has limited tolerance. Through its laws and mores society requires the family to contain sick behavior within a somewhat defined range. If the family cannot do so, there is disturbance within it as well as conflict between it and society. This conflict may not be flagrant, as when neighbors complain to the police about the sick member, but may instead be a conflict of the family's "social conscience." The thinking is: "Our son must not be allowed to expose himself; it is bad enough that the neighbors know that he is sick." Among other things, society has provided the psychiatric hospital to cope with intolerable behavior. It is a powerful representative of the demands of society. The conflicts such a family has had with society will be transferred to its relationship with the hospital and will be reflected in the family therapy situation.

When the departments of a hospital are well-integrated and joined in the common effort to help the patient and his family, additional points of leverage as well as of transferential complications are created. The points of contact may become areas of friction. In their responses to hospital policies and staff members other than the patient's therapist, families reveal their interactional peculiarities and their specific views of authority, society, and people. If the father of the patient does not want to do business in the way it is prescribed by the hospital but in the way he prefers, it is as significant as when he parks his car in the Medical Director's parking space or blocks the hospital entrance with it. Here is a chance to confront the family with its doings through other members of the hospital staff. Of course, it is important that there be ready ways of communicating such events to the patient's therapist so that he can interpret them as belonging to the family's pattern of interaction within itself as well as with society. These potentially therapeutic contacts between the family and hospital society may be called Administrative Family Therapy.

The following case illustrates how a meeting of the financially responsible family members with the Medical Director for a seemingly purely administrative purpose had a decisively therapeutic effect.

A 35-year-old acutely disturbed and negativistic but chronically paranoid schizophrenic woman had been quite a management problem in the hospital. She had an initial protracted period of improvement from acute symptoms during which she required special nursing care repeatedly. After three months the family objected to further hospitalization, indicating the financial difficulties involved. The family took the subsidence of acute symptoms as an indication that discharge could be risked, although previous hospitalizations elsewhere had rendered this assumption invalid. However, the patient's husband did disclose that his father-in-law had the means at his disposal to invest in further treatment, but would not because under the manipulation of his daughter he blamed the husband for having contributed to her illness. Thereupon the Medical Director met with the patient's parents and her husband. He pointed out that their blaming each other was of no help to the patient but enabled the patient to continue her subtle techniques of dividing them. Once the family members realized that they had become the victim of the patient's manipulations, they united and shared in the financial obligations. This enabled the patient to continue hospital treatment, with the result that considerable further improvement ensued.

Particularly in the small, analytically oriented hospital the patient population may be considered—and, in fact, often considers itself—as a "family group." This, then, is a fifth factor for consideration in dealing with family therapy in the hospital setting. The role the patient plays in this group into which he is introduced is determined by his own pathology, the composition of the patient population at the particular time and its response to him, and the program prescribed for the patient. In our own particular hospital all patients get to know each other quite well rather quickly, and know and are known by most personnel very rapidly. There is a "family feeling" and atmosphere which a patient soon senses, and relates himself to in one manner or another. He plays out his emotional and interpersonal conflicts in this intramural family.[6]

He will find various father and mother surrogates and sibling rivals among medical and nursing staff members as well as fellow patients. The fact that these persons are really different from the image the patient has of them contributes to his feelings of turmoil, helplessness and anxiety. This state leads to friction but offers the opportunity of confronting the patient with his incongruent way of relating to others, all of whom may contribute to his progress.

To some degree, then, the patient is a member of two families: the original and the intramural. These "families" are in covert or overt competition, and the patient may therefore play one against the other. Both seem to be beckoning for his loyalty. Each tries to prove it is more successful than the other in helping him improve. Each is protective that the other may not harm him. Each tests the vulnerability of the other.[7] The relatives are often anxious when the hospital is successful in the face of their own failure. They may try to impose their own views as to what is right for the patient. They may doubt their choice of hospital and question its integrity. Although High Point Hospital began family therapy partly out of sympathy for the suffering family,[8,9] this competitive trend is constantly gleaned from the remarks of physicians, nurses, and other staff members. The one who seems most prone to a competitive and critical attitude toward the family is the patient's therapist.

As mentioned above, a patient is ordinarily hospitalized when the intrafamilial or social pressures become intolerable for the family. This brings us to a sixth matter—the problem of the "identified patient." Foremost exponents of family therapy, in their attempts to treat the family as a unit, tend to disregard the identified or primary patient as such.[10-13] This seems feasible when conjoint family therapy is conducted either outside the hospital or in research with an entire hospitalized family. Once the primary patient is hospitalized, however, he unavoidably is the "identified" patient until his discharge, and this is the inescapable fact.

The question then arises whether this will undo the effort of family therapy before it has begun. Can we still observe the family as a system of interactions between the components of the system, although interaction has been restricted to the exchange of letters and contacts during visiting hours and conjoint sessions? Does the hospitalization not confirm to the remainder of the family that it is the patient's individual pathology that has to be focused upon, not the family's interactional and role pattern? Will it not tend to insulate itself and stress the patient's role as scapegoat? Does this not blatantly contradict the usual views on family therapy?

The mere fact of hospitalization does indicate the patient as the sick one. However, once he is removed from the family and injected into a dynamic setting, changes do take place for the patient and these need to be kept in mind in the conduct of family therapy. He is freed to a considerable degree from the influences that cast him into the role of a scapegoat. He belongs to an intramural family of patients whose previous roles resemble his, and of sophisticated staff members who openly call him a patient but assign a role to him which is different from his previous one. He is no longer the outstanding member in his original family where he, by virtue of his symptomatology, became the focus of the family's attention and efforts. Even the sickest patient in the hospital can no longer engulf others. This new role in the intramural family helps him feel less the burden of being the identified patient. Many other changes also take place in the patient's relationship to his family as he gathers insight about it in individual psychotherapy, and from his study of his intramural family relationships. These, too, play their part in the family therapy sessions.

The act of hospitalization affects the remaining members of the family in various ways,[14-16] which also need to be kept in mind for their own influence on conjoint family therapy in the hospital setting. The family equilibrium has been upset and new forces are unloosed within it. The original "scapegoat" is now protected by a potent group, and as he progresses he becomes a new force in the family constellation. Not only may his progress be more rapid than that of the others, but he may undergo changes unforeseen and unanticipated by them. Changes considered healthy by the medical staff may not be to the family's liking, yet the family is rather helpless because of its obligation to the therapists. It is not easy for the family to contradict those to whom they have brought their "identified" one for help. Ultimately, then, they have to turn to these very psychiatrists for guidance and growth. For many it is not a very palatable situation. Most distressing of all is the growing recognition that they must expose their own individual and collective pathology when it exists. They had expected to remain untouched. Should their pathology be too severe or the psychiatrists too unskilled, they will wreck the effort rather than relieve the "scapegoat" of his role and share the responsibility with him. Should the family be on the healthier side, a good working relationship may be established with it and a happier solution achieved.

Among the many factors which affect inpatient family therapy is the degree of illness of the hospitalized patient. As a rule, he is more severely ill than the ambulatory patient treated in family therapy. This is logical to the current trend which discourages hospitalization until there is no other alternative. Additionally, the family unit as such is more likely to be rather desperate, if not actually pathological. Facts such as these will naturally determine if, when, and how family therapy is conducted. The catatonic or flagrantly deluded patient is hardly a candidate for effective family therapy. Certainly it would be too much for other family members to sift the irrational from the rational of the patient's productions. Technically the family would first need a great deal of preorientation, and the patient a period of individual therapy to first stabilize.[17] When all are distraught and the therapist has little command of the situation, as is true initially, it would hardly be a good time to start family sessions. Such conditions require the greatest degree of flexibility, even more so than under ambulatory circumstances.

SUMMARY

Family therapy is now an integral part of our armamentarium in psychiatry. Although it is primarily used on an ambulatory basis, there is increasingly good reason for its use with hospitalized patients. However, hospital conditions are sufficiently different to warrant careful study in order to modify family therapy accordingly. Our purpose with this paper is to bring attention to some of the many factors which will affect such therapy in the dynamic hospital setting.

REFERENCES

1. Greenhill, M., Gralnick, A., Duncan, R., Yemez, R. and Turker, F.: Considerations in evaluating the results of psychotherapy with 500 inpatients. Amer. J. Psychother. 20:58-68, 1966.
2. Gralnick, A.: On behavioral determinants in a therapeutical milieu. *In*: The Dynamics of Psychiatric Drug Therapy (G. J. Sarwer-Foner, Ed.). Springfield, Ill., Charles C Thomas, 1960. pp. 227-240.
3. Gralnick, A., and D'Elia, F.: Role of the patient in the therapeutic community: patient-participation. Amer. J. Psychother. 25:63-72, 1961.
4. Lind, A., and Gralnick, A.: Integration of the social group worker and psychiatrist in the psychiatric hospital. Paper read at the Meeting of the American Psychiatric Association, St. Louis, Mo., May 10, 1963, pp. 53-58.
5. Boszormenyi-Nagy, I., and Framo, J.: Hospital Organization and Family Oriented Psychotherapy of Schizophrenia. Proceedings of the 3rd World Congress of Psychiatry, Montreal, 1961.
6. Rabiner, E., Molinski, H. and Gralnick, A.: Conjoint family therapy in the inpatient setting. Amer. J. Psychother. 16:618-631, 1962.
7. Brodey, W.: Some Family Operations and Schizophrenia. Arch. Gen. Psychiat. (Chicago) 1:379-402, 1959.
8. Gralnick, A.: Family therapy: general and specific considerations. Amer. J. Orthopsychiat. 32:515-526, 1962.
9. Gralnick, A. and Schween, P.: Family therapy. Psychiatric research report 20. Amer. Psychiat. Ass., Feb., 1966, pp. 212-217.
10. Ackerman, N.: Family therapy and psychoanalysis: the implications of difference. Family Process 1:30-43, 1962.
11. Bowen, M.: The family as the unit of study and treatment. Amer. J. Orthopsychiat. 31:40-60, 1961.
12. Jackson, D.: The monad, the dyad, and the family treatment of schizophrenics. *In*: Psychotherapy of the Psychoses (A. Burton, Ed.). New York, Basic Books, 1961, pp. 318-328.
13. Satir, V.: Conjoint Family Therapy. Palo Alto, Calif., Science and Behavior Books, 1964.
14. Lefebvre, P., Atkins, J., Duckman, J., and Gralnick, A.: The role of the relative in a psychotherapeutic program: anxiety problems and defensive reactions encountered. Canad. Psychiat. Ass. J. 3:110-118, 1958.
15. Gralnick, A.: The family in psychotherapy. *In*: Individual and Familial Dynamics (J. H. Masserman, Ed.). New York, Grune and Stratton, 1959, pp. 183-191.
16. Fleck, S.: Psychiatric hospitalization as a family experience. *In*: Special Treatment Situations, Vol. 1. Des Plaines, Ill., Forest Hospital Publications, 1962, pp. 29-37.
17. Gralnick, A.: Conjoint family therapy: its role in rehabilitation of the inpatient and family. J. Nerv. Ment. Dis. 136:500-506, 1963.

14

Transference-Countertransference Phenomena in Choice of Shock

Review of One Hundred Eight Cases, with a Comparative Study

EDWIN L. RABINER, M.D.
ALEXANDER GRALNICK, M.D.

ALTHOUGH ELECTROSHOCK is a useful treatment, we are not uniform in our thinking about it, and are often in doubt as to when and how to employ it. While certain criteria for its use have been established with respect to diagnosis, symptomatology, and chronicity, it remains difficult to predict accurately the response of any individual patient to it. This state of affairs may well be traceable to our failure to consider, in the design of studies bearing on the effectiveness of EST, the host of variables pertaining to the patient, the therapist recommending and administering EST, and the relationship of the doctor and the patient.

Over the past 15 years many workers experienced in the use of the somatic therapies have been impressed with the influence of factors other than the three enumerated above on

---

Reprinted from the *A. M. A. Archives of Neurology & Psychiatry,* April 1959, Vol. 81, pp. 517-521 Copyright 1959, by American Medical Association.

Funds for this study have been provided by the U. S. Public Health Service, Grant No. M2349. Dr. J. William Silverberg and Dr. Guy E. Leduc assisted in culling data from the records studied. Read in abbreviated form at the 114th Annual Meeting of the American Psychiatric Association, San Francisco, May 16, 1958.

the effectiveness of EST in any given case. These factors broadly fall into two categories: those relating to the total make-up of the patient, and those inherent in the treatment situation itself, including the quality of rapport established before and during the period in which EST is being administered.

With respect to the patient himself, recent attention has been given to such factors as basic character structure,[1-5] the degree of reaction on the part of the patient to his own illness,[3] and the nature of the patient's resistances.[6,7]

With regard to the treatment situation itself, Gralnick,[8] on the basis of an intensive study of the effectiveness of insulin treatment at Central Islip State Hospital, suggested that the specific value of insulin lay in its setting the stage for a very special type of interpersonal relationship. He conjectured that another drug which produced deep sleep for a few hours without lowering the blood sugar level and which would permit the same treatment procedure as that associated with insulin administration would produce equally good results. Controlled studies have borne this out for insulin[9] and ECT as well,[10] indicating the need for closer scrutiny of the psychologically therapeutic effects of the somatic therapies. Important recent studies in this area have been made by Bogen-Tietz[11] and by the Henry Phipps Clinic under Whitehorn,[12] stressing the importance of the therapist's active participation in an anaclitic role to the patient receiving EST.

The quality of the relationship established between doctor and patient, in which context the choice of EST is determined, has also received attention recently. Investigations conducted by Hollingshead and Redlich[13-17] have indicated that when diagnosis is held constant, somatic therapy is given more commonly among the lower social classes. Workers at Hillside Hospital[18] have reported that patients who differ most strikingly from their therapists with respect to cultural background are most likely to receive electroshock therapy, apparently on the basis of defective communicative interaction between patient and therapist.

Factors such as these are not usually considered as influencing the decision to employ shock. Yet if they are generally operative, albeit inadvertently, we are not giving EST entirely for the reasons we think we are. Since the effectiveness of any treatment can be judged only in relation to the reason for which it is used, the final evaluation of the efficacy of EST must await the full elucidation of all the factors bearing on the decision to use it in any given case. The present study was undertaken toward the end of identifying additional factors, recognized and unrecognized, influencing the decision to use EST.

CLINICAL MATERIAL STUDIED

This study was conducted in a 40-bed private psychiatric hospital, where each patient receives three to five hours of psychoanalytically oriented psychotherapy per week, regardless of whether EST is concurrently employed. Each patient receives a highly individualized program of treatment and management. Shock treatment is used as an adjunctive procedure, and only to the degree that it will bring a patient into sufficient contact with reality to establish a meaningful relationship with his therapist. It is not used with any predetermined idea as to number or frequency of treatments, though grand mal seizures are sought.

The decision to give shock is in all cases made by the medical staff as a group and therefore is subject to the staff doctors' individual biases toward that modality of treatment. The structure of the hospital is such that all members of the staff involved in these decisions have intimate daily contact with all the patients, including occasional interviews of them. Where differences arise among the staff as to whether proper indications exist for the addition of EST to a patient's program, the therapist's opinion is given major consideration; but the decision is made by majority vote.

The material of this study consists of the clinical records of 58 patients receiving EST plus psychotherapy and 50 patients receiving psychotherapy alone. Patients were randomly selected from among the hospital admissions of the last three years. These records contain detailed progress notes on the clinical course of the patient. Patients given shock received from 1 to 20 treatments, one-half receiving 6 treatments or less.

METHOD

The shock and control groups were compared with respect to diagnosis, presenting symptoms, age, duration of illness, and personality traits affecting the doctor-patient relationship, in an attempt to isolate factors responsible for patients falling into the shock rather than the nonshock group. The data compared with respect to diagnosis, symptomatology, years ill on admission, and age require no further explanation. Personality traits were classed as tension-producing or not in relation to their impact on the doctor-patient relationship.

The following traits, attitudes, and behavioral qualities were considered likely to produce transference-countertransference tensions: clinging, pleading, excessively dependent, demanding, and controlling behavior; manipulative tendencies; negativistic or nihilistic disposition toward therapy, and openly hostile attitudes to the therapist. The justification for assuming that these characteristics were apt to lead to doctor-patient tensions lay in our clinical knowledge of what transpired under such conditions. We had observed that they regularly produced deficiencies in rapport, the extent of which varied with their degree and the sensitivity of the therapist to them. We had often seen pleading, excessively dependent patients lose faith in the therapist who could not quickly satisfy their pleas or demands for relief. Analytic modification of these traits could not proceed well under such conditions. We had experienced discomfort in working with such patients and felt certain that this communicated itself to the patient, further impairing rapport.

In our study, then, patients were categorized as having traits impairing rapport on the basis of the multiple mention of one or more of them in the doctor's notes.

DATA

The results of this comparative study are given in the accompanying Tables.

TABLE 1.—*Diagnosis*

	Shock Group (58 Cases), %	Nonshock Group (50 Cases), %
Schizophrenic reactions	64	76
Paranoid type	36.4	50
Undifferentiated	24.2	20
Catatonic	3.4	4.0
Hebephrenic	0.0	2.0
Involutional psychoses	17.3	2.0
Manic-depressive psychoses	5.2	4.0
Psychotic depression	1.7	4.0
Organic psychoses	5.2	4.0
Psychoneuroses	6.9	10.0
Total psychoses	87.1	90.0

The groups were found to be comparable with respect to the frequency with which a psychosis was diagnosed, 87% of the shock group carrying such a diagnosis, while 90% of the control group was considered psychotic. The somewhat greater incidence of schizophrenias in the control group (76%, as compared with 64%), was offset by the heavier representation in the shock group of involutional psychoses (17% as

TABLE 2.—*Symptoms*

	Shock Group	Control
Depression	32	32
Suicidal trends	13	15
Overactivity	3	2
Delusions	17	15
Agitation	14	14
Withdrawal	4	10
Poor controls	1	0
Uncooperative attitude	7	0
Panic	1	0
Aggressive behavior	1	4
Disturbed nonaggressive behavior	7	4
Nihilistic ideas	3	0
Hallucinations	2	3
Confusion	4	7
Apathy	2	1
Unrealistic thinking	1	0
Autism	1	2

compared with 2%). Thus diagnosis correlated significantly with choice of shock only in the involutional group, but was not a factor in the other diagnostic groups comprising the great bulk of the material studied.

A comparison of the presenting symptoms of the two groups surprisingly revealed no significant differences in any of the following conventional indications for EST: depression, suicidal trends, overactivity, disturbed or destructive behavior, delusions, hallucinations, confusion, withdrawal or autism.

TABLE 3.—*Duration of Illness on Admission*

	Shock	Nonshock
6 mo.	31	16
6 mo. or more	27	34
	$\chi^2=4.34$ $P=0.0256$	

However statistically significant differences did occur when the age and duration of illness in the two groups were compared, the shock group being skewed in the direction of older patients whose illness had been of shorter duration.

With respect to tension-producing traits, it seems striking that 63% of the shock group manifested one or more such traits, as against 30% of the nonshock group. It was also of interest that of the 15 control patients who were considered for but not given shock, generally because of physical contraindications, 12 showed tension-producing traits. In general, three factors were most highly correlated with the selection of particular patients for shock treatment. These factors, namely, age, recency of onset of illness, and presence of tension-producing traits, each predicted shock at a statistically significant level of confidence whereas diagnosis and symptomatology did not. This remained equally true when the involutional patients were excluded and when schizophrenic patients alone were considered.

TABLE 4.—*Age*

	Shock	Nonshock
40 or over	30	14
40	28	36
	$\chi^2=5.32$	
	$P=0.0139$	

Based on χ^2-test determinations and Fisher's exact probability test, the presence of tension-producing traits correlated most highly with the appearance of a patient in the shock group and statistically, therefore, is the most accurate predictor of shock in this series of cases.

Clinically, as well as statistically, there is reason to believe that the tension-producing traits might be the most significant of the three factors in determining choice of shock.

TABLE 5.—*Personality Traits*

	Shock	Nonshock
Presence of tension-producing traits	37	16
Absence of tension-producing traits	21	34
	$\chi^2=8.01$	
	$P=0.00135$	

The age difference in the two groups was a matter of less than five years above or below the age of 40. On this account, it did not seem probable clinically that whether a patient was 35 or 45 would determine his selection for shock. Likewise, with respect to the "duration of illness" factor, we at our hospital generally view recency of onset as an indication for psychotherapy, rather than shock.

On the other hand, we had often observed situations in which the staff was in full agreement that indications for shock were or were not present, but the patient's therapist would disagree with the group in its decision to give or not give shock treatment. This suggested that the therapist was responding to something in the psychotherapeutic situation which he was either unaware of or unable or reluctant to communicate to the others. The presence of countertransference tensions might well account for this discrepancy of opinion.

We next attempted to study further the tension-producing group to see whether their disurbing traits appeared independently or in association with the factors of diagnosis, symptomatology, age, or duration of illness. If these traits were only a dependent variable, the factors with which they appeared might really be the determining ones in the choice of shock.

A comparative study was made only of the patients manifesting these traits; this involved 37 patients receiving shock and 16 not receiving shock. We found that in all age groups tension-producing traits are two to four times as prevalent in the shock as in the nonshock group. Further, this is equally true whether the illness is of more or less than six months' duration. No new differences appeared except for one. Of patients with these traits who received shock, 54% manifested agitation more frequently, as opposed to 25% of the nonshock group. Conceivably, this is so because agitation places a further strain on the doctor-patient relationship, makes more prominent the patient's tension-producing traits, and confronts the therapist with the need to produce relief more rapidly.

Of the 58 cases receiving shock, of which 37 manifested these tension-producing traits, in only 2 were rapport difficulties specifically cited in the record as playing a role in the choice of shock treatment. In the other 35 instances, the therapist was either unaware of the significance of these traits in his choice of treatment or felt constrained not to indicate the role they played. Yet many of the other 35 records lent themselves to the inference that transference-countertransference tensions were operative.

COMMENT

We are mindful of the fact that we are applying statistical methods to complex phenomena which are difficult to identify with certainty. However, the application to psychiatric phenomena of improved research designs, such as the double-blind study, has focused attention on the importance of the doctor-patient relationship in any treatment procedure. Currently in most instances choice of shock treatment is determined by the rather classical indications, such as diagnosis, symptomatology, recency of onset, and psychotherapeutic inaccessibility. Apparently, however, more subtle human factors may be of importance in the selection of treatment. Our study would seem to suggest that the first three indications are not necessarily as significant as had been thought, and that the fourth indication warrants more detailed study. It would seem reasonable, as this study suggests, that there are aspects of the patient-therapist relationship which influence, albeit inadvertently, the selection of shock treatment for a patient, perhaps as much as anything else.

Although ordinarily considered obscure, it would seem that such subtle human factors as tension-producing traits can be studied with some degree of accuracy. Perhaps our future studies, as well as those of others, will suggest leads for improved methods of defining and quantifying the complex factors inherent in all psychiatrist-patient relationships. It is to be hoped that shock treatment will not be completely abandoned because of our enthusiasm for the new drugs before such studies can be thoroughly done.

The objection might be voiced that our findings are specific to High Point Hospital, and otherwise inapplicable. However, it may also be that it is because of the very nature of our program that we are able to discern and validate these findings. Consequently, there is room to believe they are applicable wherever psychiatrist and patient meet in a treatment situation, whether the doctor is aware of these influences on him or not.

SUMMARY

The clinical records of 58 patients receiving electroshock and psychotherapy were compared with those of 50 patients receiving psychotherapy alone. Comparative figures in the two groups were obtained for diagnosis, symptomatology, duration of illness, and tension-producing traits with respect to the doctor-patient relationship.

Neither diagnosis nor symptomatology predicted the choice of shock in the cases studied. Recency of onset, age, and the presence of tension-producing traits with respect to rapport each predicted shock at a statistically significant level, the last being the most accurate predictor.

Attention is called to the need for further study of the subtle human factors that may operate in the selection of shock treatment for any given patient.

REFERENCES

1. Gralnick, A.: A Seven Year Survey of Insulin Treatment in Schizophrenia, Am. J. Psychiat, 101:449-452 (Jan.) 1945.
2. Gralnick, A.: A Three-Year Survey of Electroshock Therapy: Report on 276 Cases. Am. J. Psychiatry, 102:583-593 (March) 1946).
3. Pacella, B. L., Piotrowski, Z. and Lewes, N. D. C.: The Effects of Electro-Convulsive Therapy on Certain Personality, Am. J. Psychiat. 104:83-91 (Aug.) 1947.
4. Kahn, R. L., and Fink, M.: Personality Factors in Behavioral Response to EST, Confinia neurol., to be published.
5. Kahn, R. L., and Fink, M.: Prognostic Value of Rorschach Criteria in Clinical Response to Convulsive Therapy, Confinia neurol., to be published.
6. Hill, L. B., and Patton, J. D.: When Physical Therapy (Shock) Facilitates Psychotherapy, Am. J. Psychiat. 113:60-65 (July) 1956.
7. Patterson, E. S.: Psychophysiologic Resistance in Insulin Coma Therapy, J. Nerv. Ment. Dis. 125:547-557 (Oct.-Dec.) 1957.
8. Gralnick, A.: Psychotherapeutic and Interpersonal Aspects of Insulin Treatment, Psychiat. Quart. 18:179-196 (April) 1944.
9. Ackner, B., Harris, A., and Oldham, A. J.: Insulin Treatment of Schizophrenia, a Controlled Study, Lancet 1:602-611 (March 23) 1957.
10. Brill, N. Q., Crumpton, E., and others: Investigation of the Therapeutic Components and Various Factors Associated with Improvement with Electroconvulsive Treatment: A Preliminary Report, Am. J. Psychiat. 113:997-1006 (May) 1957.
11. Bogen-Tietz, E., and Jordan, J. H.: Rapid Treatment of the Psychotic Patient Integrating Electronarcosis and Psychoanalytic Psychotherapy, Am. J. Psychiat. 114:68-72 (July) 1957.
12. Whitehorn, J. C., and Betz, B. J.: A Comparison of Psychotherapeutic Relationships Between Physicians and Schizophrenic Patients When

Insulin Is Combined with Psychotherapy and When Psychotherapy Is Used Alone, Am. J. Psychiat. 113:901-910 (April) 1957.

13. Esecover, H., Jaffe, J., and Kahn, R.: Psychotherapeutic Techniques with Electroshock Patients, J. Hillside Hosp. 7:17-25 (Jan). 1958.
14. Freedman, L. Z., and Hollingshead, A. B.: Neurosis and Social Class: Social Interaction, Am. J. Psychiat. 113:769-775 (March) 1957.
15. Hollingshead, A. B., and Redlich, F. C.: Schizophrenia and Social Structure, Am. J. Psychiat. 110:695-701 (March) 1954.
16. Hollingshead, A. B., and Redlich, F. C.: Social Class and Psychiatric Disorders, in Interrelations Between the Social Environment and Psychiatric Disorders, New York, Milbank Memorial Fund, 1954, pp. 195-208.
17. Redlich, F. C., Hollingshead, A. B., Roberts, B. H., Robinson, H. A., Freedman, L. Z., and Meyers, J. K.: Social Structure and Psychiatric Disorders, Am. J. Psychiat. 109:729-734 (April) 1953.
18. Kahn, R., Pollack, M., and Fink, M.: Social Factors in the Selection of Therapy in a Voluntary Mental Hospital, J. Hillside Hosp. 6:216-228 (Oct.) 1957.

15

The Implementation of Psychoanalytic Concepts in Hospital Practice

J. WILLIAM SILVERBERG, M.D.
FRANK G. D'ELIA, M.D.
EDWIN L. RABINER, M.D.
ALEXANDER GRALNICK, M.D.

PSYCHOANALYTIC PRINCIPLES and techniques have found far less application in hospital than in office practice. There would appear to be a number of reasons for this. Some of these stem from changes over the years in the economic, logistic and philosophical considerations governing hospital practice.

Thus, prior to World War II, it was considered therapeutic to treat the mentally ill individual in a remotely placed "sanitarium" away from the noxious milieu that spawned his illness. This view, which placed no premium on rapid return to the community, was compatible with time consuming, psychoanalytic investigation within the hospital—but unfortunately there were few psychoanalytically-trained people in hospital work at that time.

Nowadays, when the psychoanalytically-trained hospital worker is not, or need not be, in such short supply, the time such workers might spend with a hospitalized patient is. That is, the greater demand for hospital beds and rising costs of

---

Reprinted from *Science and Psychoanalysis,* G. Masserman, Vol. VII, pp. 280-289, Copyright Grune & Stratton, Inc., 1964.

hospital care impel us toward briefer hospitalizations. These economic factors are reinforced by growing commitment to the idea that anything other than the briefest possible hospital stay promotes regression and fixes dysfunction. Now, as it were, that we have the trained analysts to practice the method, we are constrained by economic and philosophical injunction against its use.

We do not propose to argue here the economic problem. We do, however, advance the thesis that long-term hospitalization need not result in regression and fixed dysfunction. On the contrary, it can be the only way in which enduring improvement can be produced in the adaptive capacities of certain patients.

For such patients, the duration of hospitalization is entirely subordinate to treatment goals. If the hospital has a properly devised social structure and treatment program there need be no regression, for it need not be an inferior substitute for the patient's home. Rather, in many instances, it can be vastly superior to it and, like office psychoanalysis, can induce the development of a healthier, more mature personality than the patient has ever known.

The confines of the hospital are necessary if these patients are to be prevented from fleeing the social repercussions of their behavior before they learn from it, if they are to be prevented from isolating themselves or from recruiting kindred spirits to reinforce socially their maladaptive behavior.

Were the psychoanalyst simply to transfer his practice from his private office to the mental hospital, he might continue to see the true "therapy" as limited to the psychoanalytic treatment sessions. During the rest of the time, the patient might be seen as protected by the hospital but not as being actively treated. This would be in contrast to a therapeutic concept which embodies the idea that treatment goes on hour by hour and day by day during the entire period of the patient's hospital stay. Such a concept implies that the social structure of the hospital exerts a therapeutic influence and extends the analytic process beyond the interview situation.

Working with hospital patients, the analyst is likely to find himself at a peculiar disadvantage. His process is based on verbal communication; yet frequently the hospital patient does not utilize a verbal treatment process well. How then can the psychoanalyst's therapeutic concepts be successfully applied to hospital patients? Can the essentially verbal one-to-one process be suitably modified for the treatment of less communicative patients in the complex social structure of a psychiatric hospital?

We are suggesting that these questions can be answered in the affirmative. In addition, it is possible to evolve treatment techniques which offer the analyst more information about his patient, thus making his poor communication less of a handicap to therapy. However, modifications must be made if the concepts and process of psychoanalysis are to be implemented in psychiatric hospital practice. It is the purpose of this paper to describe some of the modifications which we have found necessary and useful.

In office practice, the analyst's field of observation is limited to what the patient tells him verbally, or indirectly by his behavior. In the hospital, the field of observation can be vastly expanded. The therapist is in a position to observe the patient directly, or through the eyes of trained observers, in a variety of activities. He receives reports from the nursing staff, activity workers, other therapists and, at times, other patients. The flow of direct observational data to the therapist enhances his knowledge of and insight into the patient. It materially reduces the therapist's dependence on the patient's own reportings in sessions. Parenthetically, it might be added that reports from other trained observers sharpen the therapist's own observations, and consensually validate or enhance his ability to detect countertransference. This involves collection of a multitude of data over a twenty-four-hour span by professional observers in several disciplines. If the hospital is small enough, and if there are enough intersecting lines of communication, it is possible for the skilled observers to develop a comprehensive grasp of the patient, as well as of the hospital dynamics. The many details about the patient and the various therapeutic and anti-therapeutic processes within the structure as a whole come under the purview so that a coherent plot begins to unfold.

As an illustration of the kind of procedure by which patient and hospital processes can be scrutinized, analyzed and synthesized, the following segment of an interdisciplinary staff conference is described.

The Conference:

It is reported that Henry, a patient, has been censured for the general untidiness of his room by another patient, who is Chairman of the Housekeeping Committee. This latter patient's doctor remarks that the censure occurred only because of personal antagonism to Henry. Dr. B., Henry's therapist, is quick to support the idea that Henry has been unfairly censured. He has been maintaining for some time that Henry has improved and that reports to the contrary are erroneous. At the previous week's conference, the staff as a whole had seen Henry's behavior as disruptive, but Dr. B. had disagreed. Now, he reiterates his contention that Henry *has* improved and that the censure for untidiness was unfair and the result of personal bias. The Director of Nursing hastens to contradict Dr. B. and to affirm that Henry is indeed untidy, constituting quite a problem to the Nursing Department. He adds that the Patient's Housekeeping Committee is functioning well and has fairly stated a purely factual finding. The conference leader, a seasoned psychoanalyst, has seen over a period of weeks the unfolding of this emotional interplay with growing conviction that Dr. B. is seriously involved in a countertransference which compromises his good judgment in the management of his patient. He points out that he has noted that Henry tends to dissociate and fall apart under stress. "Why, that's common knowledge" the social group worker points out. "When that happens, the patients all say 'that's Henry.' " But it has not been noted by Dr. B., who has a stake in his patient's "improvement." Dr. B. now begins to see that he may have been wishfully overlooking this. The conference leader then points out to Dr. B. that, because of this unrealistic investment in his patient's illusory improvement, he may find himself reacting to Henry in the future with anger when Henry fails to live up to his expectations. Dr. B's reply to this is a candid admission that he has already, indeed, begun to feel such twinges.

At the following week's conference Henry again is discussed, this time in terms of his slyly arrogant attitude toward the patient chairman of the Housekeeping Committee. Now the conference leader offers the formulation that Henry's actions suggest that he thinks of himself as playing a role other than that of a patient. By this time, Dr. B. is much more receptive to such a formulation and gives additional supporting evidence in terms of Henry's grandiose productions in individual sessions. Upon discussing some of these productions in detail at the conference, a picture of Henry emerges which suggests that he is acting out with his fellow patient his Oedipal rivalry with his father.

Particularly to be noted in this material are first, contribution by trained observers representing various disciplines and points of view; second, the psychoanalytic orientation of the conference; third, the attention to dynamics occurring within the staff as well as among the patients; fourth, the group therapy aspect of the conference particularly in its implications for resident training; fifth, the emergence of the observation that Henry is involved in the acting out of transference.

TRANSFERENCE

While many transferences occur in the daily life of the patient, they cannot be satisfactorily and meaningfully analyzed because of the absence of an objective observer. Therefore, in office practice it is only in relation to himself that the analyst can discriminate accurately between what is real and what is transferred. In this analytic model the patient verbalizes most of this material.

However, the significant past is also remembered behaviorally, quite independently of the cognitive aspects of recall. By carefully observing and differentiating what is appropriate behavior from what is not, we can catch sharp glimpses of the nature and genesis of the patient's psychopathology.

Whether by virtue of his more serious pathology, or the resistances engendered by his being institutionalized, the psychiatric inpatient is often unwilling, or unable, to comply with the fundamental rule. Thus, the communication level essential to traditional forms of self-inquiry, all too often, cannot be achieved. Handicapped, then, by a paucity of reliable verbal data, the analyst in hospital practice must draw more heavily on behavioral observations in developing understanding of his patient's abnormalities. He can do this by observing the acting out of transference in the milieu of the hospital.

The pathological behavior and attitudes rooted in the genetic development of the individual are projected upon suitable personages, as well as aspects of the institution itself. They may be observed in a wide variety of interpersonal transactions which occur in full view of the trained staff. These, then, become data equal in reliability to the information gleaned from the transference to the therapist.

The following considerations appear to be relevant to the fullest utilization of this transferential vantage point:

(1) The daily routine of the hospital must be designed to encourage interaction by each patient with other patients and staff. For this purpose it is useful that there be bound social contexts within which a wide range of functioning and patterns of behavior can be scrutinized, experimented with, and tested. The use of task oriented patient committees with fixed responsibilities to the hospital community, the strategic assignment of roommates, tablemates, committee members are useful interaction facilitating devices.

(2) Detailed accounts of his patient's interpersonal transactions must promptly reach the therapist.

(3) In order to insure that the observations reported are relatively free of bias, irrational attitudes at all staff levels

must be dealt with constantly and actively. For example, if a patient bridles at a hospital rule as arbitrary and authoritarian, it can tell us something about him, provided we are sure the rule is neither arbitrary nor authoritarian.

Case Illustration:

A young woman who seemed compelled to seek out sadistic men far beneath her social station was admitted to the hospital in a hopeless, apathetic state. In psychotherapeutic interviews, she spoke of herself as stupid, unattractive and immoral, and would say little else. Her therapist learned, through collateral sources, that she was not getting along well with other female patients of his, and was scrapping with female contemporaries while behaving in a compliant and subservient fashion to older women. Following the therapist's announcement after some months of treatment that he would be going on vacation, it was reported by other patients via their therapists, that our patient began to make sexual advances toward sicker male patients, as well as several hospital groundsmen. Even in the absence of her verbal cooperation, he was able to surmise the meaning of her pattern of self-debasing promiscuity as a response to paternal rejection. When he interpreted this to her, she replied in dramatic confirmation, "I don't care what I'm doing! You made me love you and now you're walking out."

As a corollary material to the use of the transferential vantage point, we would like to suggest an approach to dream interpretation which utilizes detailed knowledge of the patient's day to day living. This approach is applicable to the patient who reports dreams, but is unable, or unwilling, to free associate to them or help much in their interpretation. Using the reported manifest content and detailed reports of what is going on in the patient's life in the hospital, the therapist may be able to understand the unconscious meaning of the dreams. He may then either interpret the dreams to the patient, or simply use the information to deepen his own understanding of the patient's dynamics.

Case Illustration:

A twenty-two year old schizophrenic girl had developed an erotic transference to her therapist. One day she was observed to leave one of the hospital rooms angrily, when another of her therapist's patients remarked, "You know, we can share him." The patient did not tell her therapist of this incident, but Nursing reports did. The next day when the patient reported a dream, "I was smothering my sister to death," she offered no associations. Nevertheless, the likely meaning of the dream was obvious to the therapist.

COUNTERTRANSFERENCE

The phenomenon of counter transference is universal in the one-to-one doctor-patient relationship and will naturally occur in the hospital treatment situation. Its detection and resolution, however, are not universal. For the concept of countertransference is unique to the psychoanalyst, and unless psychoanalytic theory and thinking are firmly entrenched in the hospital, the chances are that it will go unnoticed and unresolved.

In general, the private practitioner works alone, and therefore, has no one but himself to detect countertransference. The hospital therapist need not depend on himself alone, because in conferences and discussions of the analytically-oriented hospital staff, there exists the opportunity for constant, mutual supervision to keep countertransference exposed and therefore at a minimum.

Relatively inexperienced psychiatrists training in a hospital will have many more countertransference reactions than their fully trained counterparts of the senior staff. Obviously, it should be part of their training to have these reactions clarified. Although some of the work of uncovering such countertransferences can be done in individual supervisory sessions, we have found it particularly useful to use staff conferences for this purpose. This is done for several reasons: First, it offers an opportunity for the entire staff to benefit from the experiences of the individual members. Secondly, the presence of the residents as a group offers them both peer support and peer validation. By the latter we mean the possibility that agreement by the other residents will overcome resistance of an individual resident to exposure of countertransference attitudes. This is analogous to the situation in group therapy where a group member can accept an interpretation by the therapist more readily, if other group members support it. Finally, when senior staff members point out countertransference among themselves, the residents are able to see the process as non-judgmental and non-critical. Mutual supervision of this sort can be done successfully only in an atmosphere of trust, where there is good understanding of, and devotion to, the treatment method and its goals. A team approach, with the various members of the team working together closely, is clearly a necessity.

Obviously, there will be differences in the types and frequency of countertransference phenomena which one is likely to observe in senior and junior staffs. Among the latter, because of their incomplete training, such reactions are frequent and often gross phenomena. Not precisely countertransference, but certainly a related phenomenon, is the acting out of a resident in relation to his patients, which is in the service of sibling rivalry with other residents or struggles against senior staff authority:

Going back to the vignette of the interdisciplinary conference, some of the points mentioned can be illustrated. Over a period of three weekly meetings, resident therapist Dr. B. became aware of his over-protective attitude toward his patient, Henry. In the course of three conferences, the combined weight of observation and opinion of the Director of Nursing, social group worker, the conference leader and the resident group overcame his resistance and clarified his countertransference for him. At the last meeting he was enabled to contribute material which helped to clarify the dynamic significance of his patient's behavior. As a postscript, it can be added that Dr. B.'s understanding was further deepened in his individual supervisory session. In discussion here, it became apparent that Dr. B., a new resident, was involved in a sibling rivalry with his fellow residents. For this reason, he had tended to identify with his own patient in the latter's rivalry with another patient, rather than analyze it.

We have stated previously the importance of assuring unbiased observational data by constant alertness to countertransference, not only in the psychiatric staff but at all staff levels. Numerically, the bulk of the staff is nursing personnel. One cannot expect from them anything like the level of psychological sophistication that is to be found in an analytically-led psychiatric staff. Nevertheless, in a stable and well-led Nursing Department, the blind spots and biases of the various members can be fairly well-known and balanced out by the head of the department. The latter is in intimate contact with the psychiatric staff so that he can participate directly in the mutual supervision and analysis of countertransference attitudes which have been described.

HOSPITAL ORDERS

"Actions speak louder than words" may be a worn cliché, but it contains two important ideas: first, that in every action there is an implied verbal statement; second, that the action is a stronger statement than the verbalization. Actions, or conditions enforced by orders, are sometimes used in orthodox analysis. A classic example is Freud's setting of a fixed termination date for the analysis of "The Wolfman." Freud noted that "eventually the patient came to see that I was in earnest" and "under the inexorable pressure of the fixed limit his resistance and his fixation to the illness gave way."[1]

It is a special condition of institutional practice that a variety of actions must be taken at the beginning of, and throughout, a patient's hospitalization. Among these are the admission procedure itself, assignment to ward and room, orders for medication, special precautions, prohibitions, and/or freedoms. These actions are generally done *to* the patient, his acquiescence being a desirable, but not a necessary condition. Carrying them out is a necessity if, in fact, the patient is to receive hospital care. However, where psychotherapy or psychoanalysis is considered the crucial treatment, there is a tendency to see these actions as outside of the psychological treatment. There is no denying, nonetheless, that the administrative and medical orders or actions, and the statements they imply, have a powerful psychological impact. If the therapist understands this, he adds an additional dimension to their usefulness and his own effectiveness.

From a psychological point of view, orders written by the hospital therapist may be said to have an impact on the patient similar to that of an interpretation, because they can have the effect of confronting him with and helping him to focus upon disordered behavior, feeling, and thinking. As noted, every order can be translated as a statement, or statements, to the patient. For example, an order increasing medication may convey the statement "you are more upset emotionally." An order increasing visiting time may convey the statement "your condition is improved."

It is not intended to imply that a hospital order and a verbal interpretation are one and the same thing. The order enforces a condition. When properly utilized it powerfully reinforces what often has been verbally interpreted to the patient repeatedly without effect. The order, or the condition which it enforces, can clarify for the patient, can arouse resistance or overcome it, can stimulate self-exploration. The order, therefore, though not precisely an interpretation, can serve an interpretive function.

Presumably, in an effort to maintain a non-directive "therapeutic" relationship and at the same time take the many necessary actions, some hospitals have set up a system in which the "therapist" treats the patient and the "administrator" directs and writes orders. However, since the so-called "administrative orders" are in fact an integral part of the patient's therapy, logic dictates that the authority to write them may only be vested in the therapist—the doctor who really knows the patient. Additionally, vesting such orders in the so-called "administrator" results in what we consider to be an unrealistic splitting of the therapeutic figure. The patient tends to see the therapist as warm and permissive and the administrator as cold and authoritarian. A more realistic "parental" figure for the patient to relate to is one who combines permissiveness and authority.

The twenty-four-hour-a-day treatment concept has been previously emphasized. An advantage of an order used to reinforce an interpretation is that, perforce, the statement it implies is said to the patient over and over again without the therapist's having to repeat it. The condition or order statement may be in force constantly, as, for example, when the patient is ordered to reside on a closed ward. When an activity such as work on the Housekeeping Committee is ordered, the meaning may be reiterated each time the patient engages in the activity.

Case Illustration:

An eighteen year-old girl was admitted in an acute schizophrenic reaction. She made a satisfactory recovery from this, whereupon her pathologically low self-esteem, lack of recognition of herself as an individual, and parasitic dependence on her parents became evident. Her integration in hospital activities was marginal. She persistently requested longer and longer visiting periods with her family, despite repeated verbal interpretations by her therapist emphasizing the connection between her complaints of inadequacy and her pathological dependence on her parents, currently expressed in the demand for longer visits. At length, he wrote an order prohibiting the patient's visits with her parents.

For a short period she expressed bitterness over this. Her behavior in the hospital remained unchanged. Then with surprising rapidity she began to assert herself. In the sessions, she moved from complaining about no visiting to exploring in a meaningful way her dependence on her parents. Gradually she began to participate more effectively in hospital activities.

The no visiting order had spurred the patient into focusing on her pathological dependency needs in her psychotherapeutic sessions. Concomitantly, removed from contact with her parents, she used the hospital environment constructively in developing new patterns of relatedness.

CONCLUSION

In this paper we have attempted to describe some aspects of a hospital treatment method which greatly expands the psychoanalyst's field of operation. In the process of so doing, an attempt has been made to define the special conditions associated with the psychoanalytic treatment of the hospitalized patient, the implications of these conditions in terms of certain key psychoanalytic concepts, and modifications of techniques which take proper cognizance of these conditions. A further implication is the responsibility of the psychoanalyst in the primary task of designing the social structure and treatment programs of certain hospitals. For if he maintains a high degree of flexibility, and is willing to accept the challenge, who is better qualified to take responsibility for the setting up of a psychotherapeutic community of this sort than the psychoanalyst?

Our belief in psychoanalysis as a treatment method, and above all as a research tool, should encourage us to see that increasing efforts are made to apply it to the residential treatment setting. The wedding of psychoanalytic theory and method to the concept of residential milieu therapy will deepen and enrich both. It offers the opportunity for thorough-going treatment of patients who could not be contained and involved in therapy in any other way.

REFERENCES

1. Freud, S.: Collected Papers, Vol. 3. London, Hogarth Press, p. 478.

16

Psychoanalysis and the Treatment of Adolescents in a Private Hospital

ALEXANDER GRALNICK, M.D.

IN THE PRESENT ERA of psychoanalysis the great debate (to which some of us have become quite accustomed) seems to have borne results. Fewer question the logic and need for traditional psychoanalysis to change its techniques, if not its basic theory. An ever-larger body of analytically trained people of various shades of opinion have taken increasing command of the psychiatric scene. Their clinical experience has been different, and they have been trained by younger teachers whose minds have been more flexible. Under these circumstances, it begins to appear that a new set of theories and practices may be crystallizing out for adoption.

More and more voices are openly raised against psychoanalysis of any persuasion. Some of these belong to highly trained, serious thinkers; others, unfortunately, to those less competent. The evidence of ferment is implicit in the newer trends in psychiatry, such as milieu therapy, group therapy, family therapy and community psychiatry, and the increasing emphasis on drug therapy. No matter how we may try to cling to old theory and techniques these practices will increasingly call up new beliefs and ways quite different from those employed in one-to-one therapy. If there is any logic to the idea that theory grows out of practice, then the

Reprinted from *Science and Psychoanalysis,* J. Masserman, pp. 102-108.

handwriting is on the wall. Modification is the order of the day.

The trend in hospital practice, too, is in the direction of great change. Witness the mushrooming of psychiatric units in the general hospitals. Quick symptom relief and rapid discharge are made of the essence. In office psychoanalytic practice six hours per week has given way to five, to four, to three and even to two. Duration of sessions has gone from 60 to 50 to 45, and even fewer minutes. "Brief psychotherapy" and hypnosis are increasingly popular. It would appear that long-term typical psychoanalytic therapy may ultimately be the field for the few die-hards, the students or the researcher. While it is true that in all these new ways the language of psychoanalysis is still used by many, it is often with meaning and intent hardly resembling their original.

In our view psychoanalysis is a part of psychiatry that deals with a particular method of understanding and treating human beings, and carries with it a theoretical substructure. More of its content, both theoretical and technical, has been applied to the study, comprehension and treatment of the emotionally and mentally disturbed, but relatively little of it to the basically normal individual. In the area of theory there are marked differences among those who consider themselves psychoanalysts, so much so that some believe the others to be pretenders. Under such circumstances communication becomes difficult, advancement is slowed, and the achievement of effective methods of treatment is delayed.

I am convinced, for the moment, that we are born with a certain constitution, and that accordingly, we react differently to environmental stimuli. We have "basic needs" for which we seek gratification, and are given gratification by others around us. In the process of being nurtured the infant takes on human qualities and a personality which depends on the nature of this constitution and the nature of the personalities of those about him. People other than those in the family have much to do with one's personality development, which itself is the result of a continuous process. We think, too, that the growing child plays a more active role in his ultimate outcome than many tend to believe.

We do not hold with beliefs in the basic nature of the "sexual drive" and the universality of the oedipus complex. They do not adequately account for personality development and psychopathology. We believe that in addition to "constitution," social forces, rather than sexual instincts and anatomic differences determine one's role and attributes.

My basic orientation has been changing during the past 15 years that I have served as the Medical Director of a psychiatric hospital. I sense that psychoanalytic colleagues in similar posts have also gone through changes in their basic thinking and find themselves favoring certain procedures they would never have dreamed of while in office practice.

I am sure that our experience with adolescents as well as adults has had a fair degree to do with the modification of our analytic thinking and practices. Twenty years ago I would not have dreamed of seeing the family of an office patient, let alone treating its members conjointly with the patient. Today we do it, and accordingly think differently about the origin and treatment of mental illness. Twenty years ago I thought that the essence of technique was to help the patient gain insight so as to enable him to change into a healthy human being. How naive! Insight is not enough! Hospitalized patients require "management," or structuring. Such a regime has a wholesome effect upon them. They seem to learn from it, particularly if it has a pattern of consistency.

Repeated experiences of this nature tell you that you cannot sit by and listen, or let the patient do as he pleases, but that you have to inject yourself into his life and thereby order and influence it. You see increasingly that this process can help him grow and change. You find, for instance, that some patients need to be forced to enter the hospital or compelled through court certification to remain there. You find that such action has a wholesome effect, that is, that something done against the patient's will does help him. This type of experience is not what one is quite accustomed to in office psychoanalytic practice. You actually get to the point with certain "acting-out" youngsters where you find yourself recommending that the court indicate that he (the patient) has the choice of going to jail or the hospital. You get a little horrified at yourself but know that otherwise the course of this youngster will continue dangerously downgrade. But again you see a patient progress with the opportunity for treatment which society has forced upon him. Hundreds of experiences of this nature are bound to change what you do, and compel you to re-evaluate your original basic theory.

Although all this may sound far afield, I do believe that the theory one holds must determine the nature of the hospital he conducts. Otherwise, he is in real trouble. Thus we believe that the social structure of our Hospital is most important to its patients. We look to it to implement our theory, and yet to put it to the test, so that it may be altered with changing clinical experience. We emphasize individual psychotherapy and give each patient three sessions per week. However, we see it as but one element of the totality of factors which have a therapeutic effect. In fact, we hold that psychotherapeutic sessions may be rendered wholly ineffective if the social structure of the hospital is not "psychotherapeutic." I have often said to the overzealous therapist who believes that only his three sessions per week are helping the patient: "I could let you see the patient in seven sessions per week and so administer this hospital that your patients would get worse instead of better." This often has a frightening, if not settling effect, upon the dedicated therapist. But yet if he need not be omniscient and omnipotent he has the relief of knowing he does not have the entire responsibility. He knows that there are other sources to which he can turn for assistance. From this he can soon see, hopefully, that the parent too is neither the entire source of the patient's difficulties, nor the sole hope for his future.

Our therapists are "active" in their individual role with patients, but are also fully active in the patients' total program. The hospital has its own system of values which play a significant role in the lives of all those associated with it, including patient and doctor.

In some way, our supposition is that "social pressures," and all that this phrase implies, contribute to the patient's ultimate decompensation. Accordingly, the logic would seem to be to this effect: that constructive or positive forces should assist in the reversal of this direction. We thus consider psychotherapy to be one of these positive forces, particularly if it is supported by legitimate theory and consistent practice. In a "healthy" environment, then, one can more easily distinguish the "healthy" from the "sick," and be more easily helped to follow a salutary direction. The function of the psychotherapist is to help the patient achieve this in the hospital setting. Teaching and learning are active components of this process.

There is a rising percentage of young in our population; there are increasing numbers of youngsters being hospitalized, and there is a rising amount of delinquency, crime, addiction and self-destruction among adolescents. However, there are problems associated with this. First, there is no uniformity of thinking about the age limits of the adolescent. While most seem to agree that adolescence starts with the onset of puberty, few agree about the upper age limits of this so-called stage of life. Some mention the age of 18 to 21, while others will go to 24, and also speak of the "adolescent" personality of the adult. We recognize, further, that many an "adolescent" is "adult" beyond his years. The culture in which the adolescent lives is also very important. Among the major problems is the fact that very few studies indeed have been done on the "normal" adolescent. The bulk of our knowledge comes from the study and treatment of the sick youngster. The unfortunate trend has been to consider their problems as typical of all young people. Additionally, I think there is a tendency to "understand" the young to the point of often overlooking the severe psychopathology which exists in many of them.

Offer and Sabshin[1] say that in the adolescent it is "difficult to distinguish health from illness or normal turmoil from pathological process." Further, they say, "The prevalent concept of adolescent turbulence does not evoke images of so called normal behavior." Anna Freud[2] writes, "Where adolescence is concerned, it seems easier to describe its pathological manifestations than the normal processes." The problem inherent in these statements is magnified further by the fact that it is extremely difficult to design a good piece of research to determine what the normal adolescent is like. However, as a beginning, Masterson[3] has made a study of 100 adolescent patients as well as of a control group. Contrary to the theorization of leading psychoanalysts, his study shows that syndromes in adolescents can be delineated and defined, and that their symptomologic manifestations are similar to the disorders of adults. He concludes that he was not dealing with disorders specific to adolescents "but rather with the usual psychiatric disorders which are appearing in this segment of the life cycle." I believe that his study supports the nature of our own observations and experience. It is important to think of these youngsters as suffering with specific disorders, and to emphasize diagnosis and treatment in keeping with them. Anything less than this can lead to delay and inadequate treatment. It is likely that many of the so-called "adolescent behavior problems" really constitute specific mental disorders. This statement is supported by the research of Masterson and Washburne[4] who also found the syndromes in adolescents may often be stable, rather than fleeting. This finding, too, is in the face of the beliefs, unsupported by research, of leading psychoanalytic theorizers that the adolescent syndromes are evanescent.

The adolescent at our hospital has the usual symptoms in various combinations seen in the emotionally disturbed adult. He has overindulged in alcohol and drugs, sometimes to the point of addiction; become underproductive in his school work or overpreoccupied with himself; paranoid in his thinking or otherwise deluded about his self-image; depressed to the point of suicidal thinking or acts; hallucinatory; or evidencing increasingly poor judgment. Anxiety and hostility in varying degrees are shown by many. "Acting-out" in the usual forms is often a thick overlay, but when examined carefully is no more than that. It is not dissimilar from the acting-out seen in adults, but in different form more appropriate to his age and opportunity.

The nature of our thinking and experience, therefore, prompts us to treat the adolescent as we do the adult. He is roomed with adults, and seated at table with them, rather than isolated to his peers. He is assigned to groups of patients, including adults in keeping with his behavior and symptoms, not his age, and given individual psychotherapeutic sessions as are adults. His daily routine is much the same as that of all other patients, and he is medicated as necessary. As he progresses we make demands on him in the "patient participation" committees in which he is placed, again together with adults. We look to the "adult" in him, and think of this as synonymous with the "rational," just as we look to the "reasonable" in the adult schizophrenic. Thus we draw on the healthier aspects of his personality. Anything less than this caters not to the "adolescent" in him so much as it does to the sick and irrational. We tend to emphasize productive and and purposeful rather than leisure-time activities.

We diagnose most of our adolescents as schizophrenics and treat them with this in mind, rather than the fact that they are young. Their problems relating to people, therefore, are more a result of this disease process than of their age, and accordingly interpret their behavior as evidence of such illness. We watch against the personality disorganization, the failing judgment, and the evidences of actual distortion of reality. The latter is really at the root of many of the "problems with authority" which are so common in adolescents. It is easily found, and early, if one sees the disease process in them, rather than their "adolescence," as accounting for their trouble.

Our treatment program is designed to evoke rather than

suppress the sick ways which patients have so that they may be known, treated and replaced by healthier behavior. Since the adolescent has more difficulties with adults than he has with peers, it seems logical to group him with adults as well as his peers. This would seem to approximate reality more, and coincide with our belief that the hospital's atmosphere should be one of "living process." The essence of our "treatment" is that we are relating to, and working and living with our patients. The adolescent patient reacts to and treats us as he has others previous to his hospitalization. The material evoked is for ready study in groups and in individual sessions. We believe, although we cannot as yet prove, that the nature of our structure and the process it permits between patients, and patients and personnel, have their own therapeutic effect.

The need for modification of psychoanalysis in the treatment of the adolescent inpatient, as well as some of the modifications we have made, have been explicit and implicit in all the above. We employ psychoanalytically oriented psychotherapy, but as one, and perhaps small, part of the total treatment process which "the hospital," in all its complexity, represents. It seems that the term "psychoanalytically oriented psychotherapy" is becoming ambiguous and warrants replacement. Perhaps the term "dynamically oriented psychotherapy" would be more appropriate. It avoids the controversy implicit in the other, and yet conveys the understanding that "process" is involved.

We believe we have designed a hospital model to implement concepts of a dynamic nature. Doctor and patient are in a dynamic relationship, on a group and individual level, which is subject to study toward the goal of helping the patient. There is room for simultaneous change in the doctor. The patient is not related to his past so much as he is to the social environment of the hospital with its own value system. The process is dynamic and directed. It involves all those associated with it in any manner—patient, doctor, relative, other doctors, nursing staff, social group workers and the variety of other personnel including the Medical Director.

REFERENCES

1. Offer, D., and Sabshin, M.: The psychiatrist and the normal adolescent. Arch. Gen. Psychiat. 9:427-432, 1963.
2. Freud, A.: Adolescence. Psychoanal. Stud. Child 13:—, 1958.
3. Masterson, J. F.: Psychiatric Illness in Adolescents: A Research Project, presented to the Society on Adolescent Psychiatry. New York, April 15, 1964.
4. ——, and Washburne, A.: The Symptomatic adolescent: psychiatric illness or adolescent turmoil. Unpublished.

17

Method of Assaying Doctor–Patient Tensions

Its Application in Assessing the Role of These Tensions in the Choice of Electroshock

EDWIN L. RABINER, M.D.
MORTON F. REISER, M.D.
WILLIAM J. SILVERBERG, M.D.
LEATRICE SCHACHT, M.D.
ALEXANDER GRALNICK, M.D.

I. INTRODUCTION

FROMM-REICHMANN, whose contributions to the application of psychotherapeutic technique to the psychoses were monumental, began her major work *Principles of Intensive Psychotherapy* by calling attention to the importance of the actual as distinct from the transference aspect of the doctor-patient relationship. An increasing recognition of the significance of this parameter has resulted from the findings of (1) collaborative studies[2-4] on mental illness by psychiatrists and social scientists and (2) more refined research techniques developed in conjunction with the evaluation of psychopharmacological agents. The as yet unmet need for methods of assessing the role of the doctor-patient relationship in clinical

Reprinted from the *Archives of General Psychiatry,* June 1961, Vol. 4, pp. 553-560.

Funds for the study were provided in part by the U.S. Public Health Service, Grant No. M2349 and in part by the Gralnick Foundation.

investigation motivated the study described herein. This is a methodological paper describing a technique for the assessment of doctor-patient tensions and its application to the study of the doctor-patient relationship as a parameter affecting the choice of a treatment agent—electroshock.

In April, 1959 we reported the findings of a comparative study of the hospital records of 58 patients receiving electroshock and 50 patients who did not receive shock.[5] The objective of this study was to identify as many of the factors associated with the choice of shock as possible by comparing the incidence of these factors in the shock as opposed to the nonshock group. The 2 groups were compared with respect to diagnosis, symptomatology, duration of illness, age, and the presence of certain personality traits bearing on the ease of relating psychotherapeutically to the patient. In the series of case records studied, neither diagnosis, with the single exception of involutional psychosis, nor the symptomatology predicted the choice of EST. However, recency of onset of illness, age, and the presence of tension factors in the doctor-patient relationship each predicted EST at a statistically significant level, the last being the most accurate predictor.

Our method of assessing relationship tensions had been crude and its reliability was untested. In addition to 22 other categories of data, record raters had been asked to list those adjectives and phrases appearing in the records which seemed to describe the patient's way of relating to the therapist and the therapist's response to the patient. From these descriptions an estimate was then made of the amount of disruptive tension in the particular doctor-patient relationship. Two discriminations were made: tension considerable or tension negligible. The significantly greater incidence of relationship tensions among the shock group seemed to invite further attention.

The present paper concerns itself with a more intensive and highly defined study of clinical records, undertaken to sharpen the focus on the subtle interpersonal factors the previous study had indicated might be operative in the choice of

EST. This study was aimed at (1) developing a more explicit, reliable procedure by which the extent of doctor-patient tensions could be estimated from clinical records; (2) testing, via this rating procedure, the finding of our previous study, namely, that the amount of disruptive tension in the doctor-patient relationship requires consideration as a significant parameter influencing the decision to give EST; and (3) developing leads for a contemplated ongoing study of the influence of doctor-patient tensions on decision making as well as on the clinical course of treated psychiatric illness.

II. RATIONALE FOR THE USE OF CLINICAL RECORDS IN ASSESSING DOCTOR-PATIENT TENSIONS

Without attempting to discriminate between personal and situational factors, the extent of disruptive tension in a given doctor-patient relationship may be conceptualized as the resultant of positive and negative attitudes of each party toward the other. Each is seen as manifesting certain specific traits, attitudes, mannerisms, and modes of relating capable of eliciting positive and/or negative feelings in the other under the circumstances attendant to their interaction.

The doctor's notes, including anamnesis, psychiatric examination, and progress notes are a running account of this interaction, reflecting through omission and commission, either deliberately and/or inadvertently the emotional interplay or feeling tone of the relationship. Although explicitly intended purely for the reporting of clinical observations about the patient, it must be assumed that these observations are contaminated to a greater or lesser degree by feelings aroused in the doctor by the patient. It can also be assumed that therapists vary greatly with respect to defensive operations used to conceal personal, nonclinical, feelings toward patients from themselves and others. One would expect these defensive efforts to be considerable in relation to material to be included in a permanent hospital record. However, since we can infer the existence of certain latent feelings from other kinds of manifest behavior, so too the doctor's latent feelings toward the patient might be elucidated through the analysis of his detailed clinical notes. Thus clinical records can also serve as potential sources of information as to the doctor's emotional response to the patient and the degree of harmony or disruptive tension between them.

In this frame of reference our rating technique was designed to direct the raters' attention in examining the doctor's notes to clues in the form of affect-laden descriptive terms, the intensity of the doctor's focus (likable or irritating), discrepancies between the apparent clinical state of the patient and the doctor's management decisions for the patient, discomfort with the patient, gratification or frustration with the patient's progress, and the degree of emotional involvement with the patient. The assumption was made that in a general way the relative frequency of positive and negative clues would reflect the emotional interplay between doctor and patient, and permit quantitative distinctions, with respect to disruptive tension, to be made between different doctor-patient relationships.

Using criteria teased out of the data of the previous study, a rating form was developed for the assessment of doctor-patient tensions as reflected in the clinical notes of the therapist. The form was designed to hold the rater to a prescribed method of examining the material, for example, by forcing present-absent judgments on a wide variety of patient characteristics. At the same time it included open-ended questions designed to elucidate in so far as possible the inferential processes by which the rater worked from the data in the record to an estimate of the extent of tension in the doctor-patient relationship.

III. THE RATING TECHNIQUE USED

The 7 kinds of information sought in the form are summarized on the following page as instructions to the raters:

1. Quote all material from the record which appears to characterize the patient's positive and/or negative attitudes

toward the doctor or which in your judgment would tend to elicit either positive feelings or feelings of impatience, hostility, discomfort, or disinterest on the part of the doctor toward this patient. Positive and negative quotations with respect to their implications for the doctor-patient relationship are to be listed separately. Similarly extract all material directly or implicitly reflecting the doctor's feelings toward the patient.

2. Complete a checklist containing 23 traits and attributes characteristic of the patient's mode of reacting to the therapist. Provision was made for discriminating between those traits explicitly described in the record and those inferred to exist by the rater. The specific items included were: clinging, manipulative, negativistic, nihilistic, sarcastic, openly hostile, depreciating, seductive, ingratiating, menacing, others (specify), intelligent, insightful, able to ask realistically for help, capacity for self-observation, accepts therapeutic leadership, acceptance by other patients and participation in the hospital program, capacity to express appreciation to the therapist, capacity to smile and be pleasant, capacity to engage in interesting conversation with reasonable flow of conversation. The first 14 items were conceptualized as tension producing with respect to the doctor-patient relationship. The last 9 were viewed as conducive to a favorable emotional field and to mitigation of the deleterious effects of tension-producing traits with respect to the therapist's response to the patient.

3. Rate on a 6-point scale going from minimal to maximal the extent to which the resultant negative traits checked in 2 would appear to challenge a therapist's clinical objectivity. This rating was considered to estimate the patient's contribution to disruptive tensions between doctor and patient.

4. Rate on a similar 6-point scale the estimated degree to which the case doctor responded emotionally rather than clinically to (3) the patient's contribution.

5. Estimate on the 6-points scale the extent of the disruptive tension in the doctor-patient relationship as indicated in 3 and 4. This rating then represented the resultant of the contributions of both doctor and patient.

6. Write a descriptive summary of the doctor-patient relationship, including an evaluation of the doctor's response in relation to the patient's mode of relating.

7. Evaluate the adequacy of each record to the task of evaluating rapport in terms of scanty, adequate, or copious.

The quotations and traits checklist (1 and 2) call for explicit material from the record. This is considered to represent the basis on which the 6-point scale estimates (3, 4, 5) are made; 5 estimates the extent of disruptive tension in the relationship; 3 and 4 attempt to estimate the contribution of each party to that tension. The descriptive summary is designed to make as explicit as possible the inferential process by which ratings 3, 4 and 5 are arrived at from the raw data of 1 and 2. Part 7 was included merely as a reflector of the detail found in the record.

IV. APPLICATION OF THE RATING FORM—STUDY METHOD

The 108 records previously studied were grouped in terms of tension levels (minimal, moderate, maximal). Ten records were chosen from each tension category to insure a sample ranging from low to high levels of disruptive tension, with the condition that 15 of the 30 record samples should have received shock and 15 not. The final sample therefore ranged from low to high tension levels although the shock and nonshock groups were not matched for tension levels. Demographically with respect to age, diagnosis, and duration of illness, the shock and nonshock groups were comparable with each other and with the parent group of 108 records described in the previous study. The group included 10 males and 20 females, which roughly corresponds with the sex distribution in our general hospital population. The 30 cases studied ranged in age from 16 to 58, mean age of the shock group being 34 and of the nonshock group 32. Ninety per cent of the cases carried psychotic diagnoses, 80% being considered schizophrenic. The one involutional patient was in the shock group.

Three raters independently completed a rating form on each of the 30 records. They received written instructions as to the application of each part of the rating form including definitions of terms used and illustrative data samples. They were told to rate only information preceding the administration of EST which in a study of the doctor-patient relationship was considered a contaminant. They had no knowledge that the study was in any way related to the choice of EST, and our previous paper was as yet unwritten. Raters of divergent backgrounds were deliberately chosen. Rater A, a practicing psychoanalyst and the former Clinical Director of High Point Hospital, had known personally all 30 of the patients whose records were considered. Six of the 30 patients had been treated by him. Rater B, a resident psychiatrist, was as familiar as Rater A with the specifics of the hospital's operation but had personally known none of the 30 patients. Rater C, a qualified psychologist, though not a total stranger to the hospital in that her husband was on the staff here for 7 years, was less familiar with the hospital's operation and also knew none of the 30 patients.

V. TREATMENT OF THE DATA

Direct quotations from the record and the trait checklist were treated in terms of the operational model, namely, that the extent of disruptive tension is the resultant of 2 resultants, each consisting of the algebraic summation of positive and negative feelings on the part of the one participant for the other. Therefore positive and negative quotes[1] and traits[2] were algebraically totaled to give quote and trait balances. We were aware at the outset that this was a highly mechanistic way to assess the feeling tone of each participant toward the other. One unit of insightfulness or ability to accept therapeutic leadership cannot be really weighted against 1 unit of excessively demanding or overtly hostile behavior. Nor can one judge the extent to which a statement in the record by the therapist, during the 12th hospital week, that the patient is friendly, cooperative and making gratifying progress, neutralizes the feeling tone connoted in the initial mental status examination by reference to the patient as arrogant, sarcastic, and unfavorably comparing the hospital therapist with her referring psychiatrist. However, we operated on the assumption that the relative frequency of positively or negatively weighed comments by the therapist in the record would reflect in a crude way trends in the emotional climate between doctor and patient.

The data were then statistically analyzed in relation to 3 objectives:

1. The reliability of the ratings in terms of inter-rater agreement.

2. The interquestion reliability in terms of the agreement between impressions gained from each of the first 5 categories of data with each other and with the rating form in its entirety.

3. The relation between each question and the choice of EST.

VI. RESULTS

1. *Inter-Rater Agreement.*—A. In Assigning Quote and Trait Scores: The quote balances on the 90 rating sheets ranged from +4 to —7 with a mean of —4. Trait balance scores ranged from 8 to —10 with a mean score of —2.

In order to test agreement between raters in assigning quote and trait scores the records were ranked for each rater from most positive to most negative quote and trait scores. Agreement among the raters in the ranking of each record was tested by the Kendall Coefficient of Concordance test, corrected for ties.

Rater agreement on all factors for which the records were rated occurred at a statistically significant level. In all cases the probability of securing this level of agreement by chance was less than one in a thousand.

This was true despite the raters' differing professional orientations, levels of experience, and familiarity with the material examined.

Gross inspection of responses to questions on which raters were not limited to a forced 6-point discrimination (i.e., items 1, 2) revealed marked disparities in the form and content of the actual data which on processing yielded such a high degree of rater agreement. As one would expect, where responses are least forced, disparity is to be anticipated and appeared in the raw data. For example, a quote rated by A as connoting positive feeling on the part of the therapist for the patient was not mentioned by B, and was seen by C as indicating negative feeling on the part of the patient for the doctor. Furthermore, the total number of quotes selected by raters of the same record varied widely (at the extreme from 13 for Rater A to 5 for Rater C).

Question 2 forced a yes or no decision from the rater in relation to 23 traits manifested or absent. Inter-rater differences for a given record were often marked, varying between 2 and 9 checks at the extreme. All 3 raters agreed that a particular trait was present or absent in a particular case only one-third of the time. Yet, with respect to both quotes and traits, they did agree at a significant level on the balance between positively and negatively charged items with respect to rapport in any given case. This suggests that differing intermediate steps in terms of the identification and weighting of cues from the records led to similar conclusions as to how doctor and patient felt toward each other.

In contrast to the detailed but unstructured information sought in 1 and the explicit, detailed but forced choices of 2, the 3 factors assessed on a 6-point scale forced 1 highly inferential response from the rater. Agreement in 3, 4, and 5 could again be seen by reference to the raw data of 1 and 2 to exist in spite of individual rater differences in categorizing and weighting specific cues from the records.

Testing the agreement of the essays (6) describing the doctor-patient relationship was totally unfeasible because of the lack of uniformity in descriptive terms used as well as aspects of the relationship emphasized. Nevertheless, they were of value in understanding the reasons for significant disagreement in questions 1-5 in the few cases where it did exist.

2. *Agreement Among Questions Asked.*—If all of the 5 ratings obtained actually reflected the amount of disruptive tension in the doctor-patient relationship, then one would expect to see a pattern of covariance among them such that patients falling above or below the median in one would do

so in all 5, e.g., patients assigned a highly negative quote balance would have a similarly negative trait balance and would be rated above the median with respect to patient contribution to disruptive tensions.

Agreement between quote and trait balance and tension scores was computed on the basis of respective medians by applying Fishers Exact test for correlated proportions. P varied between 0.05 and 0.005 in each case indicating covariance among the 5 tension factors studied at a significant level. However, the large number (one-third to two-thirds of the subjects) falling into the median category on the 6-point scales, where categories 1 and 6 were used only negligibly, indicated that although 6 categories are available, these questions do not adequately discriminate among the majority of the subjects. The significant probabilities, however, are interpreted as demonstrating significant relationship between the questions in so far as patients above or below 1 median will tend to fall above or below the median of another question, even though the median may differ from question to question.

3. *The Relation Between the Questions and the Choice of EST.*—A. Relation Between Quote and Trait Scores and the Probability of Receiving EST: For both the shock group was skewed in the direction of negativity. Using zero as the cut-off point rather than the median more sensitively discriminated between the shock and non-shock groups although a significant level of confidence in this regard was reached only with respect to quote score (A2). The greater sensitivity of the zero cut-off is probably explainable on the basis that the records were individually and not comparatively scored. Raters were therefore responding not to deviations from a group median but to absolute amounts of positivity or negativity.*

* The correlation between specific traits and the choice of shock was not statistically analyzed because of the small numbers involved. All negative traits with the exception of ingratiating and seductive were encountered more frequently among the shock group. There were 6 times as many

TABLE 1.—*Tension Scores and EST*

Tension Score	Patient Tension Factor EST	Patient Tension Factor No EST	Doctor Tension Factor EST	Doctor Tension Factor No EST	Relationship Tension Factor EST	Relationship Tension Factor No EST
1	0	0	0	3	0	1
2	0	5	10	10	2	7
3	8	6	2	1	4	6
4	3	4	2	1	6	1
5	4	0	1	0	3	0
6	0	0	0	0	0	0

B. Relation Between 6-Point Scales and EST (Table 1):

Table 1 indicates a skewing in the shock group toward higher tension scores for each of the 3 tension factors. The median record falls into Category 3 for the patient and relationship factors and Category 2 for the doctor factor. Choosing the median as the cut-off point, the relation between above and below median category of the 6-point scales and EST is given in Table 2.†

The 6-point scale data therefore indicate that scores above the median in both the relationship factor as well as the patients' contribution factor predict shock at a statistically significant level, the former being the more accurate predictor. The doctors' contribution scores showed the least variability and the lowest median, suggesting that the training and maturity of the therapist form a cushion against excesses of positive or negative feelings toward the patient. Nevertheless, a trend is apparent in the direction of higher tension scores for the doctor in cases receiving EST. When the 3 tension

---

ratings of menacing in the shock group, 3 times as many ratings of nihilistic, pleading, and clinging, twice as many ratings of hostile and sarcastic, with the other negative traits showing mere pluralities. Patients rated as ingratiating were evenly divided in the shock and nonshock groups. A rating of seductive was found 3 times more frequently in the nonshock group. Among the assumed positive traits "accepts therapeutic leadership" characterized the nonshock group 2½ times more frequently than the shock group. Pluralities favoring the nonshock group occurred with respect to capacity for self-observation, insightful, able to ask realistically for help, intelligent, and capacity to smile and be pleasant.

† The fact that N is less than 30 in each table results from the omission of subjects falling in the median category.

estimates are totaled for each patient, scores greater than the median significantly predict EST ($p = 0.05\text{-}0.02$).

TABLE 2.—*Relation Between Above and Below Median Category of the 6-Point Scales and EST*

Relation to 6-point scale median	Patient Tension Factor EST	Patient Tension Factor No EST	Doctor Tension Factor EST	Doctor Tension Factor No EST	Relationship Tension Factor EST	Relationship Tension Factor No EST
Less than median	0	5	0	3	2	3
Greater than median	7	4	5	2	9	1
	p=0.05		p=N.S.		p=0.005	

Rating 5, the estimated tension in the doctor-patient relationship represents the target determination. All others were included only to enforce a uniform rating procedure and to make as explicit as possible the process of arriving at the relationship tension estimate (5). The fact, however, that relationship tension estimates predict shock more accurately than any of the 4 subfactors on which it is presumably based suggests that the inductive process of the rater has not been sufficiently explicit by the rating forms. To put it in other terms, the whole is a more sensitive indicator than the sum of its parts or than any of its parts individually. The quantifying of doctor-patient tensions by the raters involved the use of cues from the material that they have not been able to specifically identify within the limitations of this rating technique.

With respect to the adequacy of the individual records (7) to the task of evaluating the doctor-patient relationship no significant correlations were found between rater estimates of adequacy and the interrater agreement, interquestion agreement, or relationship of tension to choice of EST.

The application of this rating procedure to a clinical record requires between 30 and 45 min. per rating.

VII. COMMENT ON FINDINGS

Our findings then indicate that by following a relatively uniform and explicit examination procedure multiple observers can make reliable estimates from hospital records as to the relative proportion of positively and negatively charged relationship clues, as well as of positive and negative traits in the patient, with respect to their impact on the emotional field characterizing the doctor-patient relationhip. Raters can also reach excellent agreement when asked to quantitatively estimate the amount of tension in the doctor-patient relationship and the relative contribution of each party to it. This is so despite differences in determining whether a particular trait is present or absent or whether a particular incident or comment as described in the record reflects positive or negative relatedness. Furthermore, subjects falling below or above the median for one of the above named factors will fall correspondingly below or above all the medians suggesting that the various portions of the rating form are influenced by a common factor, presumably one that is characteristic of the specific emotional field characterizing the doctor-patient relationship.

Our findings indicate that classifying patient tensions on a 6-point scale results in a clustering about the median, thereby affording little in the way of discriminatory criteria for the median group. However, with respect to the relationship tension factor one-third of the subjects fell below, at and above the median, respectively. For subjects above and below the median, statistically significant predictions of shock or no shock were made, so that despite its insensitivity at the median range, such a 6-point scale permitted useful predictions to be made in two-thirds of the cases.

VIII. COMMENT

Our findings suggest that clinical records can furnish reliable as well as useful information about the doctor-patient relationship with respect to reciprocal feelings and attitudes, conscious and unconscious, of the participants. Although the procedure described is probably a bit cumbersome for wide employment, it appears by virtue of its reliability to represent a feasible research tool.

In terms of methodology in assaying the reciprocal feelings and attitudes characterizing the specific doctor-patient relationship, it seems highly important that we were able to achieve excellent agreement on the balance of positive and negative clues despite specific item disagreement. This suggests that the simplicity of the technique used is deceptive and that the true state of affairs is that the balance agreement stems from implicit inferences that either cannot be made more explicit or were not because the explicit information obtained was only partially complete. It is in relation to the finding that item disagreement produces rating scale agreement that the methodological frontiers appear to lie. If scales alone were used, reliability would be good but there would be great uncertainty as to the explicit process of its attainment. Open-ended questions on the other hand, while making the operational procedure more explicit, lack comparability and therefore reliability.

The ability to reliably determine whether disruptive tensions between doctor and patient are negligible or considerable in any given case would appear to have important potential value in our quest to better understand the role of relationship factors in treatment results. In any clinical study in which the emotional interplay between the doctor and patient can be expected to be a relevant variable, methods of the kind described herein are badly needed.

The knottiest problem in devising evaluative techniques toward this end is that of holding contamination of data studied to a minimum. In this regard the worst possible technique would be one involving direct observation of the doctor and patient during interviews. Using rating forms to evaluate the doctor-patient relationship in an ongoing study might be expected to have somewhat less of an effect upon the relationship studied than rating relationships during supervision. The use of clinical records for this purpose, although it has certain obvious limitations, seems to present the most negligible contamination risk because it is retrospective. However, once it is known by the doctor that his records will be so used the usefulness of this technique might well be reduced.

Our findings also demonstrate through the use of a somewhat more explicit and reliable measuring tool than was available in our previous study the previously reported finding that doctor-patient tensions represent an oft-times overlooked determinant in the choice of EST. Because it is but one among a group of factors influencing the decision to use EST, one would not expect a linear correlation between the amount of disruptive tension and the incidence of EST but rather that the tension factor would be relevant mainly at the extremes, and would contribute less when it was close to neutral. This expectation appears to be reflected in our finding that the tension factor does not predict shock in the median range.

The suggestion has of course been made by others[6,7] that determinants of the choice of EST may include countertransference acting-out on the part of therapists, including the doctor's becoming confused and/or anxious about the course of therapy. Comment on this thesis would not be justified on the basis of our findings, since our data do not reveal the specific determinants of the observed extremes of disruptive tension between doctor and patient.

Similar studies of doctor-patient tensions as a parameter influencing the choice and effectiveness of other modalities of treatment including drugs, intensive psychoanalytic therapy, milieu therapy, etc. would appear well worth doing.

High Point Hospital, Port Chester, N. Y.

REFERENCES

1. Fromm-Reichmann, F.: Principles of Intensive Psychotherapy, Chicago, University of Chicago Press, 1950.
2. Stanton, A. H., and Schwartz, M. S.: The Mental Hospital, New York, Basic Books, Inc., 1954.
3. Hollingshead, A. B., and Redlich, F. C.: Social Class and Mental Illness, New York, John Wiley & Sons, 1958.
4. Caudhill, W.: The Psychiatric Hospital As a Small Society, Cambridge, Harvard University Press, 1958.

5. Rabiner, E. L., and Gralnick, A.: Transference-Countertransference Phenomena in Choice of Shock, A.M.A. Arch. Neurol. Psychiat. 81: 517-521 (April) 1959.
6. Wayne, G. J.: Some Unconscious Determinants in Physicians Motivating the Use of Particular Treatment Methods, with Special Reference to Electroconvulsive Treatment, Psychoanal. Rev. 42:83-87 (Jan.) 1955.
7. Abse, D. W., and Ewing, J. A.: Transference and Counter-Transference in Somatic Therapy, J. Nerv. Ment. Dis. 123:32-40 (Jan.) 1956.

18

The Future of the Mental Hospital: A Perusal of the Determinants

ALEXANDER GRALNICK, M.D.

THIS PANEL COULD LEND itself to an exercise in wishful thinking or a challenge to prophesy. Rather than do either, I prefer exploring those factors and events which will *influence* the nature of the mental hospital.

Primarily, the future mental hospital will depend on the discovery of a cure for mental illness. Were a really effective treatment to come on the scene tomorrow, one may well imagine what effect this would have. Second, the nature of such a cure would determine the ultimate hospital. For instance, were the breakthrough to involve the painstaking process of depatterning the patient's personality through some new way of relating to him, the mental hospital would be different from what it would be if the cure were physiological. Third, the future mental hospital would seem to depend on a more certain and universally agreed knowledge of the origins of mental illness. Fourth, the number of doctors and allied professionals we attract to psychiatry will have an effect on the future hospital.

The amount of money made available for research will also determine the future mental hospital, as will the areas in which such money is concentrated. I think it is fair to say

Reprinted from *Mental Hospitals: Journal of Hospital and Community Psychiatry*, July, 1962, copyright American Psychiatric Association. One of four papers read at the panel "The Future of the Mental Hospital" of the Milwaukee Divisional Meeting of the American Psychiatric Association, November, 1961.

that the bulk of research funds today goes for physical and biochemical studies. Studies which deal with the origins and treatment of mental illness in terms of human relationships are relatively neglected. Of course, where this money comes from, whether from Federal, state, or local levels or large private insurance funds, will affect the future mental hospital. How much initiative will be left to the practitioners of private hospital psychiatry may have more of a bearing on the future of the mental hospital than one at first easily sees. If events permit the survival of the private hospital, its relationship with the public institution will play a role in evolving both their futures. The extent to which there is common understanding, exchange of learning, and recognition of the mutuality of both their responsibilities and problems, all of these, plus the extent to which each can serve as a model for the other, will help mold the future mental institution.

There is no foretelling what increase we may see in the incidence of mental disease from the emotional tensions people bear in the present unsettled world. Never have so many lived so constantly under the threat of physical destruction. Annihilation is no longer a distant or foreign event reserved for others. Should the next decades show a marked rise in the number of mentally disordered the effect on the future mental hospital will not be wholesome.

No one who is tempted to peer into the future should do so without looking into the mirror of the present. Currently we see a surge of emphasis on short-term hospital treatment, which we like to feel is better for our patients. However, we have devised no method of measuring this and no one can predict the ultimate outcome for these patients. Should they return to hospitals and be less responsive to present methods of care we may yet regret our flush of enthusiasm. From some quarters we do hear that patients are relapsing at an increasing pace. No matter what our attitude about short-term treatment, however, I think we agree that the future course these patients take will contribute to the evolution of our hospitals.

Insurance plans are bound to affect the future mental hospital. It is a fact that they have affected general hospitals. Therefore, psychiatrists must play an influential role in drafting plans so that they offer the widest choice of hospital care, rather than herd patients to any single type of treatment facility, such as the psychiatric unit of the general hospital. Any undue emphasis on one type of facility is bound to narrow range and quality of hospital care.

Generally, psychiatrists are either too pessimistic or too optimistic in their public pronouncements—a little too dramatic rather than realistic. The public image of us would be a lot healthier if we made the public aware of our limitations and shared with it the fact that we are groping. To the extent that our image improves, to that extent will the public support our recommendations for the future mental hospital, and accept the patients we send into the community, the community role the psychiatric hospital wishes to play, and its own role in entering our institutions to help and be helped by us.

The movement of population to suburban areas will also affect the mental hospital. The present cry is that public mental hospitals are too far from teaching centers. Even at this moment such contentions are not universally true. These hospitals are and will increasingly be contiguous to and the center of burgeoning communities. The latter bring with them the needed professional people to staff hospitals properly. Under such conditions the large state hospitals, rather than the medical schools and university teaching hospitals, may become the real centers of psychiatric care and education in the community. At that, new medical schools may actually locate in these presently suburban, soon to be urban, centers.

If I were to crystal gaze at all, I would say that it is unlikely that the large public hospitals will change radically in size in the next 25 to 50 years. Size alone is not a bar to good treatment and accomplishment, which depend on many other conditions. Decentralization into smaller treatment and administrative units within the larger whole may very well occur, rather than the common establishment of new small hospitals substituting for the old. What is ultimately to become of the large mental hospitals will depend on our basic attitudes toward them. Essentially, they are communities in themselves. If regarded and treated as such and converted into healthier communities, their patients will be exposed to a healthy type of resocialization. After all, we do not condemn towns because they are large, nor find cities unhealthy on the criterion of size alone. It is the manner in which they are governed that determines their wholesomeness.

The future should clarify and improve the relationship between public and private hospitals, particularly if the latter carry an even larger share than they already do of first admissions to institutions. Few of us realize that private hospitals, exclusive of psychiatric units in general hospitals, admit 75,000 to 100,000 patients per year—a major percentage of those admitted to all institutions. It would seem, therefore, that we need to work out better lines of communication between public and private institutions.

Since the psychiatric units of general hospitals are equipped only for relatively short-term care, we will have to improve liaison between them and the private hospitals which are geared for the longer-term care many patients require. For obvious reasons we would want to see as many as possible of those patients who require it go from these units to the private rather than the public hospitals. In this connection the nature of insurance policies has a bearing on the mental hospital and the type of care rendered patients in the future.

STUDIES NEEDED ON INFLUENTIAL FACTORS

In summary, I would suggest that consideration be given increasingly to a study of those factors bound to influence the future mental hospital. Our awareness of and ability to decide them will determine our power to predict and mold the future hospital to its best ends. Our efforts need to be directed toward evolving methods and techniques of treating the larger number of people to the best advantage. Both public and private agencies should be enlisted and encouraged to do treatment, training, and research. Organized psychiatry should take the helm and gather community support about it through the many public organizations which already exist to serve the general welfare. I think, too, that in the midst of all our efforts we should remember that as psychiatrists our main desire is to defeat the disease which is mental illness. The problem it presents our nation is of a different order from the disease itself. As doctors we are primarily interested in conquering the disease. Let us remember, therefore, that lowering the census of state hospitals and maintaining patients on an ambulatory basis are not equivalent to curing the disease. These issues should not be confused, no matter how sympathetic our attitude in alleviating the tremendous economic burden the states bear. There is no reason to believe that the patient quickly returned to the community is better off in the long run. No studies prove this. On an ambulatory basis, too, the patient is subject to much less controlled treatment and study. The ambulatory patient is not necessarily the healthier one, nor does he necessarily stand a better chance to achieve long-term compensation.

Our zeal to change the nature of hospital care may be but one step removed from thinking that mental hospitals should ultimately disappear from the scene. This has already been indicated in the literature. This approach is simply to discard the old and tried in the face of a new idea or method. As such it is part of an unhealthy tendency in psychiatry, no doubt the result of the frustration of our best efforts and intentions. The disease we treat, however, is as old as mankind, and its onset in the patient is slow, insidious and often mysterious. On this account alone we need to take the long view in considering the future of the mental hospital, which is, after all, but one of the avenues we will explore on the road toward the ultimate cure of mental illness.

19

The Private Hospital: A Promising Facility for Psychiatric Education

ALEXANDER GRALNICK, M.D.

IN 1959 THE AMERICAN MEDICAL ASSOCIATION reported there were 750,000 psychiatric beds in the United States, of which 15,000 were maintained by 296 private hospitals. These private institutions received forty per cent of the relatively acute and potentially recoverable first admissions. Private hospitals admitted 77,000 patients while all state hospitals admited 180,000. These figures indicate the tremendous proportion of early cases available in private hospitals for training psychiatrists.

Private hospitals render many services besides treating patients. Their staffs are engaged in mental health education projects, conduct psychiatric courses, are active teachers in medical schools, and render service to courts and social agencies. Many train nurses, attendants, industrial leaders, and clergymen. Accordingly the psychiatric resident is exposed to the breadth of experience which the staffs of private hospitals thereby possess.

Next to treating patients there is no more useful purpose the psychiatric hospital serves than the training of psychiatrists. Good training arises from the opportunity to actually treat patients under adequate supervision and guidance. It includes the chance to observe a variety of cases and the

---

Reprinted from *Mental Hospitals: Journal of Hospital and Community Psychiatry,* Sept. 1962, copyright American Psychiatric Association.

occasion to treat some intensively over a period of time. Our challenge is to include these facets, necessary academic education plus the specialized areas of psychiatry, in a three-year period for accreditation.

Very few single institutions can by themselves offer the necessary training program sufficiently comprehensive to gain approval. They may do so only through adequate affiliation with other institutions. Many large public institutions are unaccredited. Even some of the finer accredited programs of universities have inherent limitations despite the complex of units within them. Certainly, few private hospitals can offer a three-year program without outside affiliation.

ACCREDITED HOSPITALS TO SHARE FACILITIES

What can we do with the unaccredited public and private hospitals, and with those insufficiently accredited, to make full use of their training potential? All have much to offer, yet their facilities go to waste for unremedied reasons. Many of these are within easy reach of each other. Their staffs are colleagues and on the staffs of both the public and proprietary hospitals. What will be their fate should they ultimately be required to have a three-year program? Would not then our shortage of psychiatrists be aggravated?

Private hospitals have traditionally devoted themselves to the early recognition of problems and have taken the lead in their solution. Some nonproprietary hospitals have already developed three-year training programs and have established affiliations with public institutions. However, most private hospitals are proprietary, and it is for them now to lend their support to this movement. Each unaccredited hospital should strive to establish a qualified program for approval. Those proprietary hospitals with accredited programs should offer their clinical facilities and staffs for the training of psychiatrists in unaccredited public institutions to help the latter achieve accreditation. The exchange of experience could only result in better-qualified young psychiatrists.

The inherent problems could be solved once there is a meeting of the minds. Open-staff proprietary hospitals could set aside service beds so that their residents may have patients to treat. Members of the senior staff using such a private hospital's facilities could be required to teach these residents. The private institutions could consider establishing a "closed staff" policy which permits only the residents to treat patients, but under very close supervision. The objections to this are obvious, but residents can do a very adequate job. It may be noted too that such practice is already common in a number of nonprofit private hospitals. From the point of view of revenue, fees in such hospitals are not inconsiderable, and both the public and profession accept this situation without criticism.

More creative ideas along these lines will surely occur to those versed in the field. At the moment, for instance, our own institution, with co-operation from the New York State Department of Mental Hygiene, is attempting to expand a two-year accredited program to a three-year one. Our resident would spend his first year in a New York State Hospital and his last eighteen months at our proprietary hospital. If we are successful in enlisting the support of a medical school or other public institution, the resident would spend the remaining six months of his three-year stint there, where he would be trained in neurology and psychosomatics and would gain experience in a psychiatric unit of a general hospital. One sees in this proposed program the potential co-operation of at least three different agencies. The resident benefits from a comprehensive experience with both public and private patients treated for short- and long-term periods.

Private psychiatric hospitals offer a varying training experience. Many of them are accredited for only one year. Would it not be feasible for them to establish joint programs with the exchange of residents so that three-year comprehensive programs may be established? In this way private hospitals, both proprietary and nonproprietary, could join hands in taking leadership for the common good and for the development of superior training programs.

There are complex problems which would present themselves in any such planning. Some of these are related to traditional ideas, others to the profession's emotional attitudes toward "the private practice of hospital psychiatry," and still others to the so-called "public image" of the private hospital. Fault lies, too, with those associated with private hospitals themselves. Their thinking would also bear scrutiny. The complicated nature of these problems is matched by the organizational and economic ones.

Most patients are in public hospitals, and prevalent belief is that exposure to quantity of clinical practice is the keystone of training. The movement to university centers grows from two sources: one, the belief that all teaching naturally belongs there, and two, the belief that the solution to psychiatric illness lies in understanding the basic sciences and theories of behavior gained in the "academic atmosphere." A fundamental conflict is raised, namely, which is more important, clinical practice or understanding of the basics? Where is the emphasis most deserved? We in private hospitals must be sensitive to the effect on those bound by tradition of any attempt on our part to invade, as it were, their teaching territory. Simultaneously, those associated with present training tradition should be mindful of their own reactions.

Although we live under a system of private enterprise with profit as an underlying incentive, and although psychiatrists are engaged in office practice for private reward, two facts are self-evident: one, most psychiatric patients are supported by public funds, and many psychiatrists earn their livelihood thereby; two, there is an ingrained rejection of the idea that one should profit from the care of the sick, particularly the "pitiable" mentally ill. Regardless of the merit of the emotional attitudes implied, we need be mindful of the public effect of any movement on the part of private hospitals (particularly, the proprietary ones) to band together to advance the general welfare in an effort which at the same time would inevitably advance their own prestige.

UNITING TO ADVANCE TRAINING

Psychiatrists associated with private hospitals, particularly the proprietary ones, have a psychology of their own to explore. Those oversensitive about the position in which they have been cast may be too defensive. Defensiveness impairs objectivity, creativity, and progress. There is no reason or place for it here. Further, some may be too "ruggedly individualistic." This may account for their not having as yet joined forces to advance training programs and may be more of a deterrent force than the costs involved. There are many supporting forces, and the time is increasingly propitious for such a movement, particularly in light of the Joint Commission's calling for the development of smaller treatment units. The private hospitals have always been small, and their staffs are best equipped to lead the way in developing adequate training programs appropriate to such units.

The tangible problems involved in establishing jointly sponsored training programs are no doubt difficult. These include organization, administration, and financial considerations. However, they would not be insuperable in the face of determination and good will. Once these are present no difficulties should be insoluble.

The cost of care has steadily taken an increasing amount of state budgets. Evidence indicates that it costs the state as much to care for a patient in an active treatment unit as it does to care for him in a private hospital. The improvement of training programs will add to costs. For the private hospitals this would be no inconsiderable item, because prohibitive fees ultimately could be disastrous. Wherever warranted, could not public agencies finally lend support to qualified private proprietary hospitals prepared to enter into co-operative endeavors to expand psychiatric training? Aid could take the form of grants, fellowships, and support for building programs. Proprietary hospitals could limit the amount of income derived from such sources of help. Inasmuch as they render a service to the public, could we not aid them as we ordinarily do other private enterprises which supply a public service?

SOME IMPELLING QUESTIONS

Could we not think of proprietary hospitals as "public corporations" privately controlled and designed to give public service? Would those now in control of the proprietary hospital be prepared to think in these terms of limited income? Would those in state and Federal agencies in a position to grant aid meet such hospitals half way? Is there sufficient flexibility among us to loosen the bonds of tradition in these areas? Is the unhealthy "public image" of the proprietary hospital all of its own making? Or is it now something of a myth which is perpetuated by others for less than objective reasons too? Certainly, a new approach would help the cause of better psychiatric training.

Psychiatric training programs, whether in private or public hospitals, render several services. First, they help the public by supplying it a treatment service. Second, they serve the profession by training individual doctors to join its ranks, and the public by equipping the doctor to treat its members in hospitals and private practice. Third, a training program elevates the academic atmosphere of the hospital and thus redounds to the patient's benefit. Fourth, it serves the hospital's senior staff by sharpening its teaching talents.

The private hospital has certain inherent advantages germane to the subject of psychiatric training. It emphasizes intensive active treatment and a total therapeutic service. It is small and compact, permitting quick and adequate communication between resident and senior staff. It often concentrates on a specialized branch of psychiatry, or a highly refined method of treatment. It has flexibility of program and a minimum of "red tape," allowing prompt attention and treatment.

Private psychiatric hospitals have several responsibilities with regard to psychiatric training. They are: one, to provide training facilities and programs to meet the demand for more and better-qualified psychiatrists; two, to establish the highest-quality treatment program, which thereby demonstrates to its residents the finest example of patient-care; three, to accomplish the above and yet keep fees within the means of a fair proportion of the public fortunate enough to afford it (their needs and rights are no less important than those of the less fortunate); four, to be mindful of the large share of the total treatment load they carry, and their burden to contribute to the preparation of young psychiatrists to continue to care for it; five, to establish models of training programs as they have similarly developed model treatment plans; six, to lead the way, particularly as we face a future in which the smaller hospital will be emphasized; and seven, to be alert to the problems which will arise when smaller institutions become the desideratum, as a result of the recommendations of the Joint Commission.

Means must be found to educate the public, the profession, and governmental agencies in the importance of improved training, and the role that private hospitals play in this area. Governmental agencies, the psychiatric profession, and the private hospitals themselves have the obligation of changing the "public image" of the private as well as public hospitals. As this is accomplished, their co-operation in forging more and better training programs will be increasingly feasible. Certainly, the general welfare will be served as the private hospital is enabled to fully fill its functions to treat patients and train psychiatrists.

20

Integration of the Social Group Worker and Psychiatrist in the Psychiatric Hospital

ALICE LIND, M.S.
ALEXANDER GRALNICK, M.D.

THE INTEREST of professional workers in defining the concept of the therapeutic community and its ramifications provides the impetus for this paper. It is a report of the most recent steps in the development of a more structured and substantial psychotherapeutic community programme at High Point Hospital. The hospital treats 45 private patients and stresses, in addition to psychoanalytic psychotherapy, the therapeutic use of the hospital as a community. In so doing, it is mindful of the statement of the Expert Committee on Mental Health of the World Health Organization that "the most important single factor in the efficacy of the treatment given in a mental hospital appears to be an intangible element that can only be described as 'atmosphere.'" However, we must ultimately describe the tangible and definable qualities of "atmosphere" if it is to be understandable to others and our work is to have a scientific base. This paper is also a step in that direction.

Our approach is founded on the belief that borderline and decompensated psychotic patients reconstitute most ef-

---

Read at the Meeting of the American Psychiatric Association, St. Louis, Mo., May 10, 1963.

fectively in the process of learning to deal rationally with reality. We assume that sufficient exposure to a structured and "healthy experience" with others more stable than the patients themselves assists in producing their recompensation. This "learning" can be promoted by the planned use of the social structure of the hospital. In this sense is the hospital a psychotherapeutic community. It may yet be found that such a social structure, properly applied, actually promotes the same achievement of insight and the same type of "working through" that the doctor-patient relationship does. After all, the healthy citizen develops without the "insight" ordinarily associated with one-to-one psychotherapy. He learns and profits, and develops accordingly, from the everyday living experience to which he has been exposed. And so, the "healthier" the social structure of the hospital, the greater the opportunity to reverse the sick pattern. We realize, of course, that there are other factors yet unknown which also contribute to the process of recovery.

Patients at High Point are grouped at four levels, depending on their ability to use hospital opportunities to permit the fulfilment of their potential. Each group represents a different level of demand for adequate behavior and constructive interrelationships. The following is a description of each group: Group I: Withdrawn patients who can contribute only physical presence to a group activity; Group II: Patients who are able to simply circulate in a group with only minimum demands made for give-and-take relationships; Group III: Patients who with some help are ready to become involved around a common activity; Group IV: Patients who are better integrated but who still demonstrate strained and unsatisfactory relationships.

The assumption underlying our therapeutic group work is that the ego-building devices employed by the social group worker with normal individuals can be modified in work with disturbed ones by intensified individualization and less emphasis on fulfilment of the group goal itself. Programmes for all groups are planned primarily to meet the overall needs of the participants for help in socialization. Mutual support is achieved through shared activities and the planning for them. Techniques involve the consciously directed use of the group experience for personal growth.

This paper will focus on one aspect of this programme, namely, the integration of the social group worker and the psychiatrist in the Patient-Participation Programme.[2] Patients in Groups III and IV are assigned to participate in the six specific task-oriented committees of the hospital, namely: Housekeeping, Garden and Greenhouse, Library, Entertainment, Arts and Crafts and Newspaper. Each committee has detailed assignments geared toward a contribution to total patient well-being and the general welfare. Each committee meets once a week with a full-time staff psychiatrist who acts as adviser to the group. In addition, members of Group IV meet twice weekly to discuss problems of the Patient-Participation Programme, hospital morale, welfare and special activities. The hospital's orientation is that the therapist-adviser should have the opportunity to deal directly with the patient in individual treatment, but also to observe and handle his participation in a group. This technique furnishes the therapist a chance to be involved in more aspects of the patient's hospital life than he would if his practice were limited to individual therapeutic sessions.

It had been noted that the psychiatrists were aware of the psychodynamics and the individual conflicts manifested in a group situation. They experienced difficulty, however, in being therapeutically effective in an interpersonal situation resembling a fuller social experience. The ability to direct the patient into more helpful patterns was handicapped not merely because of counter-transference problems, but rather by lack of skill in dealing with people on this level. The psychiatrist's limited exposure to group-work programme techniques and principles lessened the effectiveness of the group experience for all its participants. In addition, awareness of the group process, the formation of cliques and other group phenomena were areas frequently unrecognized. It was interesting to note too that despite the very comprehensive planning for each of these committees, the all too common complaint of the patient in the mental hospital of "nothing to do" was still present. The medical staff considered the situation thoughtfully and recognized that some additional assistance was necessary. The problem, however, was the kind and quality of leadership to provide. It seemed important to select someone who would serve as an adjunct to the therapist in his work with the group, since the value to both the therapist, as a group adviser, and the patient, as a member of the group, was already well established. The worker introduced should be able to work effectively as a member of the treatment team and yet not interfere with the balance between patient and therapist.

After careful study, it was agreed that the addition of an experienced social group worker, serving in a working as well as teaching capacity to the staff, might be one way to cope with this problem. Initially, the group worker attended the group meetings of the committees as an observer to orient herself to the groupings, assess the level and potential for leadership of the different therapists, and to plan directions for more meaningful patient-participation. The worker was careful not to confuse or minimize the therapist's role as adviser to the group. Ultimately, she could discontinue her attendance at the weekly meetings and proceed to work directly with patients and advisers outside of the group meetings.

The integration of the social group worker with the psychiatrist required a mutual exploration for new levels of understanding, improved communication and the pooling of resources. The social group worker had joined the treatment team to add a new dimension to the psychiatrist's understanding of groups and the potent force of their processes as supporting factors in the recovery of patients. The psychiatrist, on the other hand, had much to offer in advancing the range of the social group worker in understanding the unconscious dynamics underlying the sick behavior of particular patients. Nevertheless, both the therapist and group worker seemed to approach the new alliance with a questioning frame of mind.

A weekly staff meeting set up specifically to discuss the patient-participation programme provided communication channels for two areas, namely, the therapist's report on committee functioning and the group worker's observations about particular patients, group dynamics and directions. When appropriate, the group worker used the staff meeting as the vehicle of evaluating and evoking discussion on the techniques of leadership employed by a particular therapist as he described his committee's functioning. Frequently, it was more advisable to approach the question individually outside the meeting.

The therapist-adviser sought out the social group worker to discuss aspects of the committee functioning which puzzled him, and to reflect on his own functioning in a particular committee meeting. He would enlist the group worker's aid with individual patients and evaluate the therapeutic effectiveness of particular group assignments to them. As a new patient was assigned to participate in committees, his therapist also consulted her to plan an approach in line with treatment goals. At such times, the group worker would learn in more detail the patient's successful achievements prior to hospitalization, his familial and peer relationships and presenting pathology. This professional exchange was vital to planning therapeutically appropriate assignments for patients.

The therapist's one-to-one experience has not equipped him to focus as readily on the group as a whole as on the individual patient. He seems unprepared to deal with the multiple transferences within the group in which the patients take on helping, but sometimes obstructive roles. It is important, therefore, to help the therapist integrate his knowledge of the dynamics of individual behavior with concepts of social processes. The initial tendency was to fill roles in relation to one individual at a time. It soon became clear to the therapists, however, that the interactions of a collection of patients (their problems, strengths, and weaknesses) created the uniqueness of a particular group. The therapist-adviser learned that he could not understand the group merely because he knew the stage of regression or the specific nature of each patient's illness.

The problem of leadership was another major area for assistance to the therapist-adviser. It was important to help him recognize that despite his position with patients, and his level in the hospital hierarchy, he was not "the leader" of the group. His role, instead, was to support the members in their attempts to secure the leadership position, or to accept a different role when more appropriate.

The assignment of patients to specific committees now is planful. The selection of patients to compose a committee always involves the thinking of both the therapist and the social group worker. In this way, we have been able to develop groups with members who are spotted along a wide range of behavioral adjustment. Groups are weighted on the side of health as much as possible so that the less integrated patient is encouraged and aided to rise to a higher level of expectation and functioning.

When a patient is prepared for committee participation by his therapist he is told that it is part of the treatment plan so that he may test and strengthen his social skills. Both the group worker and psychiatrist help the patient realize that he has the therapeutic advantage of moving into a more difficult social context while he is still in the protective environment of the hospital. In the therapeutic sessions, he then can explore his adjustment to the greater demands made upon him and his related emotional problems. Patients have recognized and accepted the social group worker's participation in this programme, both as a result of the therapist's reference to her helpful role and their own experience. Her observations, as well as those of the therapist-adviser, are funnelled to the treating doctor, both individually and through the regular staff conferences. Such integrated communication in a structured setting aids the "working-through" of the patient's pathological behavior. Team-work of this nature aids the diagnosis of a situation, the timing of interpretations and the understanding and evaluation of the working-through process. It spurs the quicker and fuller engagement of the patient in therapy as he is confronted in present context with the reactions of others to his behavior. These, after all, are not the reactions only of patients, but of significant authority figures often judged to be models of stability and mental health.

In one instance, Miss C., 51 years of age, an agitated, paranoid, angry and seclusive lady upon admission who had become sufficiently improved, was eventually assigned as chairman of our Entertainment Committee. This assignment necessitated very close working relationships with other members of the committee. Miss C. was ambivalent, pleased with the recognition given her by the Medical Staff, but very articulate as she described her upset with what seemed like an impossible situation for her. She pleaded to be relieved of the task. The social group worker spent a great deal of time supporting, reassuring and materially assisting Miss C. in her functioning as chairman. Miss C. used the worker as a sounding board for her doubts, anxieties and misgivings about her social acceptability. These, in turn, the group-worker transmitted to the patient's therapist. Jointly, they decided, with Medical Staff approval, that the patient be continued in the assignment. Many gains followed from this further exposure. In one evening activity, when she had delegated responsibility for the record player to another member of the committee who was relaxing in the lobby, Miss C. approached the worker and asked her to help her use "the right approach" with the other patient so she would not antagonize her. The worker's focus was on the healthy aspects of the ego function with constant emphasis on reality, learning, maintaining healthy interests and relationships.

The mental patient frequently evaluates himself as a failure in his personal relationships and functioning. The combined efforts, therefore, of the group workers and psychiatrist are bent toward helping such a patient experience and accept a feeling of success for the small to complex responsibilities he assumes during his hospitalization. A recent report from the chairman of our Entertainment Committee included the following: "The evening was very enjoyable to a great many patients, and I grudgingly admit that I felt a feeling of pleasure at seeing the groups enjoy themselves because of something I had planned and the committee had successfully and co-operatively carried through."

The example of Miss C. mentioned above is demonstrative of Fleck's[1] point of view—one with which we are in sympathy: "This does not mean total push therapy, but a good deal more sophistication and tact in one's everyday dealings with such patients. Simple exhortation will not do. Usually the ambivalent patient has received an overdose of exhortation before he arrives at the hospital. Schizophrenics need interpersonal experiences which counteract their difficulties. This requires an environment of people who reach out to the patient, who are untiring, as well as psychologically sophisticated in their efforts to engage him and who make him feel accepted despite his peculiarities but not because of them. In this connection it is important to emphasize that the uncritical acceptance of craziness, of immature demands, or so-called permissiveness is not helpful to patients."[1]

The psychotherapeutic community at High Point Hospital is structured to afford a maturing emotional experience for the patient in his many hospital relationships. It is clearly recognized by "administration," therefore, that the administrative structure of the hospital affects the quality of the role-fulfillment of staff members both as individuals and as members of a treatment-team. The quality of relationships among staff members in turn profoundly affects the quality of their relationship with patients. Our goal in working with hospitalized patients is to help them towards better interpersonal adaptations. This needs to be based on realistic and appropriate perceptions of self, of others and of self in relation to others. Consideration must then be given to the potential for meaningful and supportive interpersonal relationships that exist in the total hospital community. Accordingly, the emotional atmosphere and social milieu at High Point are under constant examination. This is evidenced by discussions at staff meetings and explorations by outside experts purposefully engaged to study the structure and patterns of interaction.

The social group worker has found "administration" and staff most receptive and co-operative and is aware that this factor has been extremely important in her effective performance. Functions of the various disciplines on a hospital staff frequently overlap and are not always clearly defined. The social group worker must be clear about the contribution her skills can make to the primary goal of the hospital and consciously integrate them into the total psychotherapeutic program. Her knowledge and understanding can also be extended to other personnel. She can cooperate with other professional services in planning and conducting orientation programs to reinforce mutuality of purpose for all levels of hospital personnel. She can interpret the theory and practice of social group work to the hospital and community at large, through a demonstration that the patient can be supported in his improvement as he participates in groups.

CONCLUSIONS

The sheltering shield of a group and a warm, accepting, but firmly structured small hospital community seem to have helped our patients lay aside defences that had previously "protected" them from painful anxieties. Accordingly, they are enabled to master these anxieties in a healthier fashion. The team approach, which considers both the one-to-one psychotherapeutic and broader social experience of the patient, increases the patient's depth of human contact. It advances the psychotherapeutic effectiveness of a patient-participation program. Additionally, it permits the fusion of the psychiatrist's training and understanding in individual pathology with that of the social group worker's awareness and skill in utilizing the social strengths still functioning in the patient.

Patients respond to this approach by becoming more realistically responsible and more involved in the treatment program, both social and individual. Therapists become increasingly aware of groups as such with their internal processes, emotional overtones and external influences. Under the conditions outlined, participation in a group is a more meaningful and satisfying experience. It seems to build confidence as well as give a real sense of accomplishment. It is further reflected in a vital quality throughout the psychotherapeutic community. The interchange, balance and feedback of both disciplines give a more complete picture of the patient's functioning. Problems of withdrawal, inappropriate behavior and acting-out, are handled more effectively. We believe that patients involved in this type of program learn new social skills and healthier ways of handling human relationships which are applicable in their post-hospital lives. These surpass their previous adaptational adjustment. It is tentatively concluded that the effectiveness of this approach warrants a review of the current collaborative rather than integrated use of the social group worker in psychiatric hospitals.

REFERENCES

1. Fleck, S.: "Residential Treatment of Young Schizophrenics." *Connecticut Medicine,* June 1962, 26, 369.
2. Gralnick, A., and D'Elia, F.: "Role of the Patient in the Therapeutic Community: Patient-Participation." *American Journal of Psychotherapy,* 1961, 15, 63-72.

OTHER AVAILABLE PAPERS

PUBLISHED

"Useful Techniques in the Treatment of Patients with Schizophrenia or Borderline States" by Mervyn Schacht, M.D. and Stephen W. Kempster, M.D., Psychiatry: Journal for the Study of Interpersonal Relations, Vol. 16, No. 1, February, 1953.

"The Technique of Employing Doctor-Patient Transactions in Psychoanalysis" by Mervyn Schacht, M.D., American Journal of Psychotherapy, Vol. VII, No. 4, pp. 653-663, October, 1953.

"Factors Determining the Initial Effect of Hospitalization on Cases of Schizophrenia," by Alden B. Starr, M.D. and Alexander Gralnick, M.D., F.A.P.A., American Journal of Psychotherapy, Vol. IX, No. 2, pp. 243-252, April, 1955.

"Strangulation of a Diaphragmatic Hernia as a Complication of Electric Shock Therapy," by Berchmans Rioux, M.D. and Alexander Gralnick, M.D., F.A.P.A., American Journal of Psychiatry, Vol. 112, No. 6, December, 1955.

"Heroin Addiction in a Male Adolescent: Complications During Psychotherapy," by J. Berchmans Rioux, M.D., American Journal of Psychotherapy, Vol. X, No. 2, pp. 296-321, April, 1956.

"Erythremia (Polycythemia Vera) As a Complicating Factor in Electric Shock Therapy: Case Report" by William F. Gibbs, M.D. and Alexander Gralnick, M.D., F.A.P.A., The Psychiatric Quarterly, April, 1957.

"Possible Synergistic Action of Chlorpromazine, Reserpine and Frenquel. A Preliminary Report," by J. William Silverberg, M.D. and Alexander Gralnick, M.D., F.A.P.A., The American Journal of Psychiatry, Vol. 114, No. 2, August, 1957.

"Hospitalization" by Mervyn Schacht, M.D., "Schizophrenia in Psychoanalytic Office Practice," Grune and Stratton, Inc., 1957.

"Psychotherapy and Adjunctive Means in Psychiatry: Case Presentation and Discussion," by William V. Silverberg, M.D., L. Clovis Hirning, M.D. and other members of the staff of High Point Hospital, American Journal of Psychotherapy, Vol. XII, No. 4, pp. 760-771, October, 1958.

"Relation of the Family to a Psychotherapeutic In-Patient Programme," by Alexander Gralnick, M.D., F.A.P.A., International Journal of Social Psychiatry, Vol. V, No. 2, pp. 131-135, Autumn, 1959.

"Problems of the Patient in Transit from Hospital to Community," by Alexander Gralnick, M.D., F.A.P.A. and Robert H. Duncan, M.D., in "Mental Patients in Transition," by Greenblatt, et. al, published by C. C Thomas, Springfield, Illinois, 1961.

"The Therapeutic Community and Its Benefits," by Alexander Gralnick, M.D., F.A.P.A., Indian Journal of Psychiatry, Vol. 2, No. 4, pp. 179-182, October, 1960. Reprinted in Diseases of the Nervous System, Vol. XXII, No. 6, June, 1961.

"Psychosomatic Aspects of Hyperadrenocorticism Treated with Chlorpromazine," by Noble A. Endicott, M.D. and Alexander Gralnick, M.D., F.A.P.A., Diseases of the Nervous System, Vol. XXII, No. 12, December, 1961.

"The Family in Psychotherapy," by Alexander Gralnick, M.D., F.A.P.A. in "Individual and Familial Dynamic," edited by J. H. Masserman, M.D., New York, Grune & Stratton, 1959, pp. 183-191. Reprinted in The Psychiatric Quarterly Supplement, Part 2, 1962.

"Conjoint Family Therapy: Its Role in Rehabilitation of the Inpatient and Family," by Alexander Gralnick, M.D., F.A.P.A., The Journal of Nervous and Mental Disease, Vol. 136, No. 5, pp. 500-506, May, 1963.

"Private Practice of Psychiatry: A Symposium" by Mr. Robert L. Robinson, Charles H. Brown, M.D., Max Rinkel, M.D., Wilfred Dorfman, M.D., Alexander Gralnick, M.D., F.A.P.A. and Jesse Arnold, M.D., The American Journal of Psychiatry, Vol. 222, No. 12, June, 1966.

"Leadership Effect on the Staff Conference Process": Leatrice Schacht, M.D. and Murray Blacker, Ph.D., Archives of General Psychiatry, Vol. 20, March 1969, pp. 358-364.

"The Problem of Primary Change in Psychotherapy and Psychoanalysis: Repair vs. Reconstruction" by Maurice H. Greenhill, M.D. and Alexander Gralnick, M.D., F.A.P.A., Excerpta Medica International Congress Series No. 150, Proceedings of the IV World Congress of Psychiatry, Madrid, 5-11, September, 1966.

"The Adolescent Inpatient: Treatment Considerations and Report on Ninety-Two Cases Compared with Ninety-Two Adults"; Alexander Gralnick, M.D., F.A.P.A., Edwin L. Rabiner, M.D., Guillermo del Castillo, M.D. and Daniel Zawel, M.S., Mental Health Services for Adolescents, Proceedings of the Second Hillside Hospital Conference, Edited by Sol Nichtern, M.D., Publisher, Frederick A. Praeger.

"Recent Considerations in the Broad Spectrum Treatment of Inpatient Schizophrenia," by Frank G. D'Elia, M.D. and Alexander Gralnick, M.D., F.A.P.A., The Journal of Psychotherapy, July, 1968.

"Social Forces and Patient-Progress in the Psychotherapeutic Community": Alexander Gralnick, M.D., F.A.P.A. and Frank D'Elia, M.D., International Journal of Social Psychiatry, 1968.

"Recovery From Near Death Associated with Phenothiazine Therapy": Case Report by Gershon Yelin, M.D. and Alexander Gralnick, M.D., F.A.P.A., Diseases of the Nervous System, vol. 29, pp. 702-704, October 1968.

UNPUBLISHED

"The Psychiatrist as Administrator in the Psychotherapeutic-Community Hospital": Alexander Gralnick, M.D., F.A.P.A. and Frank D'Elia, M.D. (Accepted for publication by Hospital and Community Psychiatry), (Read May 29, 1967 at the Menninger School of Psychiatry, Topeka, Kansas).

"Five Hundred Case Study in a Private Psychiatric Hospital: Further Considerations in Evaluation," by Alexander Gralnick, M.D., F.A.P.A., Rustu Yemez, M.D., Faruk Turker, M.D., Peter Schween, M.D. and Maurice Greenhill, M.D., F.A.P.A. (Accepted for publication by the Psychiatric Quarterly).

"How Size Affects the Efficiency of the Psychiatric Hospital": (Read at the Annual Meeting of the Central Neuropsychiatric Hospital Association March 16-17, 1963, Chicago, Ill.) by Alexander Gralnick, M.D., F.A.P.A.

"Problems of the Proprietary Psychiatric Hospital Affecting Patient Care," by Alexander Gralnick, M.D., F.A.P.A. (Read at the Annual Meeting of the National Association of Private Psychiatric Hospitals, January 17-19, 1966).

"The Effective Use of the Social Group Worker's Skills in the Dynamic Psychiatric Hospital," by Alice Lind, M.S.W. (Read at the Annual Meeting of the Central Neuropsychiatric Hospital Association, March 17-18, 1966).

"Common and Contrasting Aspects and Problems of the Proprietary and Voluntary Psychiatric Hospitals," by Alexander Gralnick, M.D., F.A.P.A. (Read at the Annual Meeting of the Central Neuropsychiatric Hospital Association, Chicago, Ill., March 17-18, 1966).

Index